# THE
# JUICE DIET

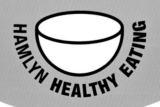

HAMLYN HEALTHY EATING

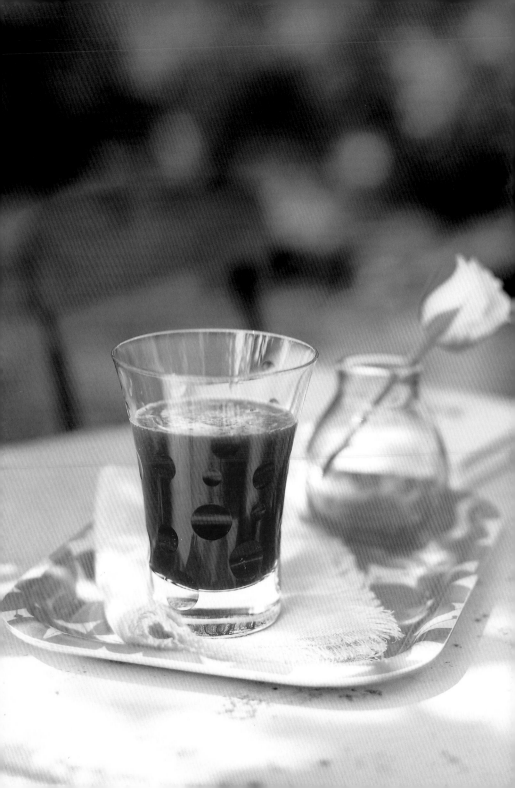

Lose 7 lbs in just 7 days!

# THE
# JUICE DIET

AMANDA CROSS

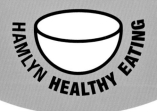

HAMLYN HEALTHY EATING

An Hachette UK Company
www.hachette.co.uk

First published in Great Britain in 2008 by
Hamlyn, a division of Octopus Publishing Group Ltd,
Endeavour House
189 Shaftesbury Avenue
London
WC2H 8JY
www.octopusbooksusa.com

This edition published in 2014

Distributed in the US by
Hachette Book Group USA
237 Park Avenue
New York NY 10017 USA

Distributed in Canada by
Canadian Manda Group
165 Dufferin Street
Toronto, Ontario, Canada M6K 3H6

This material was previously published as
The Miracle Juice Diet.

ISBN 978-0-600-62986-3

Printed and bound in China

10 9 8 7 6 5 4 3 2

**NOTES**
Standard level spoon and cup measurements are
given for the recipes.

**DISCLAIMER**
This book is meant to be used as a general reference
and recipe guide to aid weight loss. However, you
are urged to consult a health-care professional to
check whether it is a suitable weight-loss plan for
you before embarking on it.

While all reasonable care has been taken during the
preparation of this edition, neither the publishers,
editors nor the author can accept responsibility
for any consequences arising from the use of this
information.

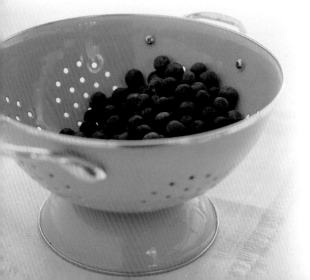

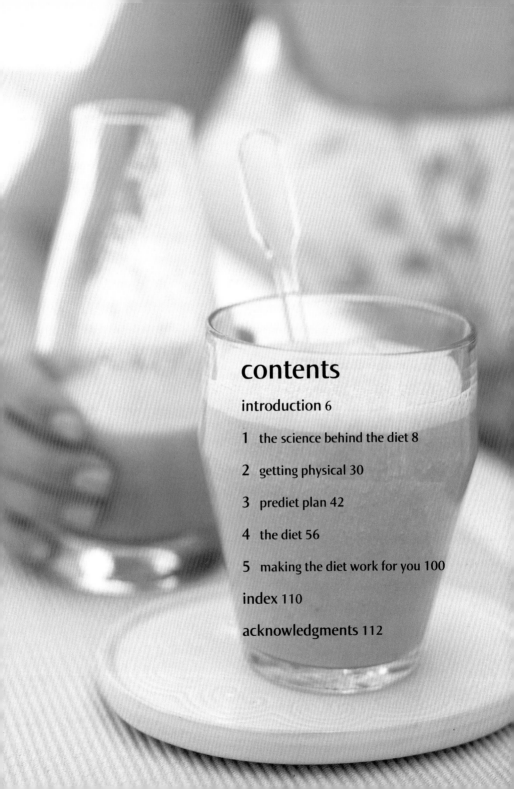

# contents

# introduction

I would bet that what prompted you to buy this book was the statement "lose up to **7 pounds** in **7 days**." Well, it's not a fake promise. You can. Whether you want to fit into a special outfit, **look great** on the beach, or jump-start a long-term weight plan, one week on the diet will help you **achieve** your goal.

It will also leave you feeling cleaner and more energized, because not only does it help you lose unwanted pounds, it will start to help your body rid itself of toxins that make you feel lethargic and set you up for a whole host of chronic conditions and diseases. Even if you are treating this as a quick-fix solution to a long-term weight problem, you will lose the pounds and give your body a vacation from all your usual bad habits. Hopefully, you'll come out the other side sufficiently inspired to improve your diet and clean up your act on a more permanent basis.

But remember—this will take determination. Making juices and smoothies five times a day takes a lot more effort than throwing something in the microwave or ordering a pizza. If you don't have a juicer and blender already, it means a little investment on your part. And although this diet isn't as extreme as other "fruit-and-vegetable" fasts, it is still a powerful detox, and you will need to make preparations so that this diet is as safe and effective as possible.

Read on: Even if you are tempted to skip the information at the beginning of the book and go straight to the diet plan, please don't. It is important that you understand the impact this diet plan will have on your body and follow the advice regarding the days leading up to the diet and exercising during that period.

Equally important is the advice on page 106 on how you should reintroduce food into your diet after your week on juices is up. I have taken into consideration how difficult a program like this can be for busy people and have allowed for adaptations that may not produce such a dramatic weight loss result, but will nevertheless allow you to lose weight steadily and revitalize your body.

Along with the dietary advice, I have suggested an exercise plan that will jump-start your metabolism and strengthen your body, as well as given tips on how to make sure your seven-day experience is as holistically beneficial as possible.

So get ready to fill your refrigerator with loads of healthy vitamin- and mineral-packed fruits and vegetables and begin your juicing journey. Destination: 7 pounds lighter.

What are you waiting for? Remember, the only person holding you back is you!

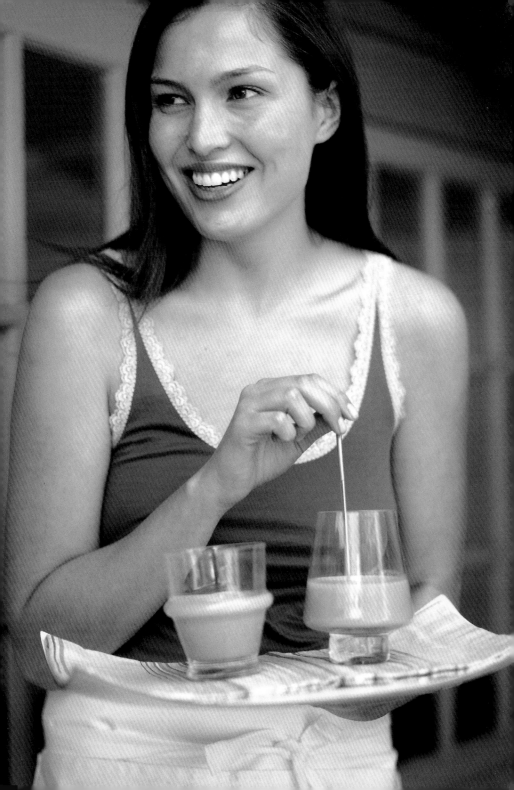

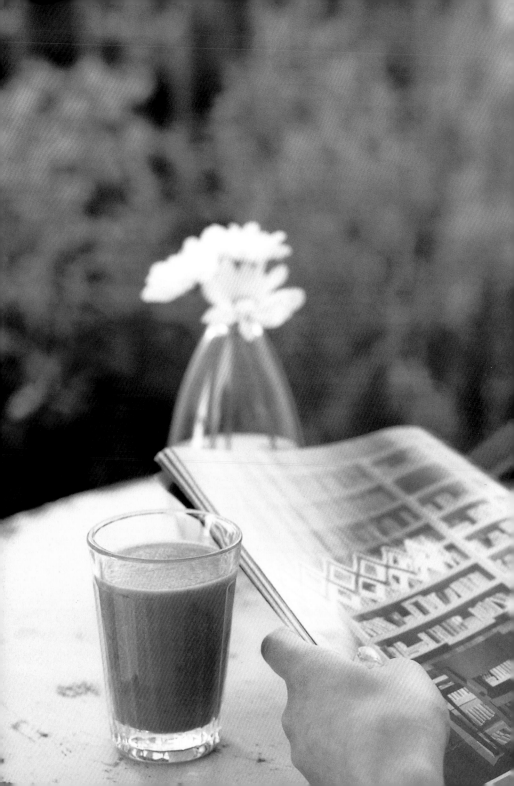

the science behind the diet

# how does the diet work?

Ever done a spring clean? Gone through every closet and cabinet in the house, **chucking out** accumulated **clutter?** Think of how much "lighter" you felt when you were done.

Your body works in a similar way. Many people carry excess weight because their systems are weighed down with an overload of toxins from poor diets and the pollutants we face daily. In addition, if you don't drink enough water, your body retains fluid in an attempt to dilute these toxins and support your vital organs. The result? Weight gain.

## the fat factor

According to studies by the U.S. Environmental Protection Agency, more than 400 chemicals have been found in human tissue—the majority of which are found in the blood, the liver, and adipose tissue—commonly known as fat.

## how does this affect your weight?

Let's look at basic biology. Various systems in your body work together to keep you "on the road" and functioning, and to do this, they all need fuel. When the quality of the fuel (air, water, and food) is contaminated, they have to work even harder, because the body has no natural mechanism to deal with man-made toxins.

Initially, the major responsibility rests with the liver. If the liver is overtaxed and unsupported by the right kind of nutrients, something has got to give, so the job goes to the excretory system. If the kidneys can't deal with the deluge of toxins in the blood, they send the toxins via the lymphatic system to a safe storage unit—your fat cells.

The more toxins your body has to deal with, the more fat cells it needs to store them, so a vicious cycle begins. As the body is burdened with more waste products, the slower your metabolism becomes, which can make losing weight a difficult task.

This diet works because it eliminates toxins in two ways: by cleansing your system and then by nourishing it, so that you quickly get a cleaner, thinner body.

## cleansing

Juices have a high water content, so they will "sweep" through your body fast, hydrating the cells and helping your kidneys and lymphatic system to rid it of accumulated waste and toxins that create the fluid retention and make you sluggish and bloated. They will also help to improve elimination from the colon and prevent the reabsorption of toxins back into the system.

## nourishing

The juice and smoothie recipes, along with the snacks and supplements in the plan, are specifically designed to support and reinforce your systems with a supercharged cocktail of nutrients essential for health and vitality (see pages 18–19 for more about vital nutrients). When you juice, your machine takes all the hard work out of digestion, because it extracts the fiber from the fruits and vegetables. This allows for their health-boosting nutrients to be absorbed immediately by the body. Your system can function more efficiently, improving your metabolism and speeding up weight loss (see page 12).

It's important when on any diet to consume enough calories. Too few and your body, programmed for survival, will think that it needs to protect itself from starvation and will store energy in the form of fat. This diet is designed so that you get just the right number of calories to be sure that you have all the energy you need for daily life and enable you to lose weight.

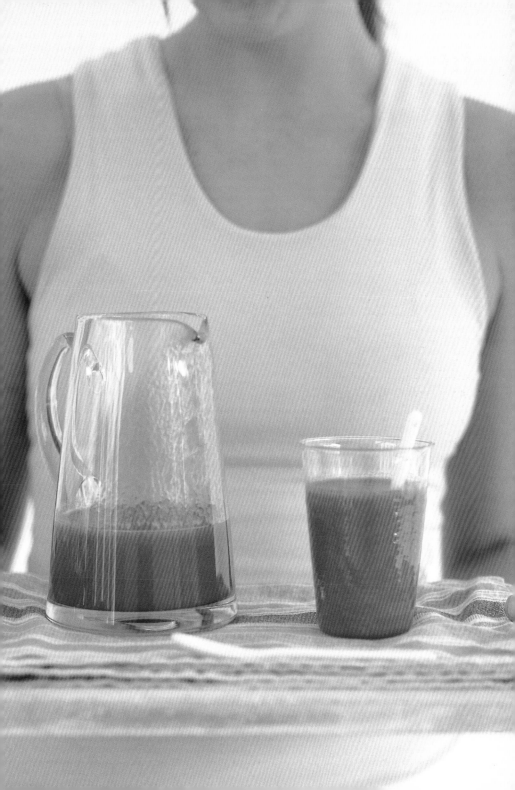

# benefits of the juicing diet

Some people will look at this diet and dismiss it as some kind of **dangerous fast**. The very same people probably drink copious amounts of coffee and alcohol, have **erratic eating** habits, and fill themselves with **unhealthy foods** that deplete instead of nourish their bodies.

Fasting generally means that you are abstaining from food, denying your body any form of nutrition. However, all the juices in this diet are full of vital nutrients that support your system and supply sufficient calories to provide your body with enough energy for your daily commitments. They also taste great, so you're not exactly depriving yourself.

The main benefits are the high vitamin and mineral content and the presence of essential phytonutrients and amino acids that ensure optimum health. They also contain vital enzymes that are responsible for the digestion and absorption of food into your body, converting foods into body tissue and enabling the production of energy. Without such enzymes, your metabolism cannot function at its optimal rate. Enzymes cannot exist at temperatures higher than 237°F, so cooking destroys many of these important nutrients.

The single most effective way to take in as many of these enzymes as possible is to eat the majority of your fruits and vegetables raw.

## why juice?

Have you ever tried to eat a whole bag of carrots? Juicing good-quality fresh fruits and vegetables gives you a huge boost of nutrients that are easily assimilated by the body because you have taken away the majority of the fiber that slows down this process. By treating your body to these highly nutritious cocktails, you will feel more sated for longer than you would if you had eaten, say, a chocolate bar high in refined sugar and unhealthy fats, which will leave your body craving for more after the initial sugar rush has worn off.

## but don't we need fiber?

Of course we need fiber, and you will be getting fiber on the seven-day plan: first, in the form of soluble fiber that juicing doesn't remove, and second, in the recommended daily fiber supplement through flaxseed and psyllium husks (see pages 24–25). It is more effective because the essential nutrients are separate from the fiber and remain immediately available to nourish the tissues and cells of the body.

## can't I just buy prepared juice from the supermarket?

Many commercially available juices and smoothies have been diluted with water, treated with heat, and may contain additives to prolong their shelf life, thus minimizing their nutritional benefit. It is best to make your own or go to a juice bar, where juices can be made to your specification with fresh ingredients right there in front of you. Alternatively, if you are stuck, seek out good-quality juices and smoothies from the refrigerated produce section.

Remember that this is a seven-day plan; on a more long-term basis, supplementing a healthy diet with freshly squeezed juices and smoothies will ensure you receive your daily minimum quota of five portions of fruit and vegetables and help provide all the key nutrients you need for maintaining vibrant health.

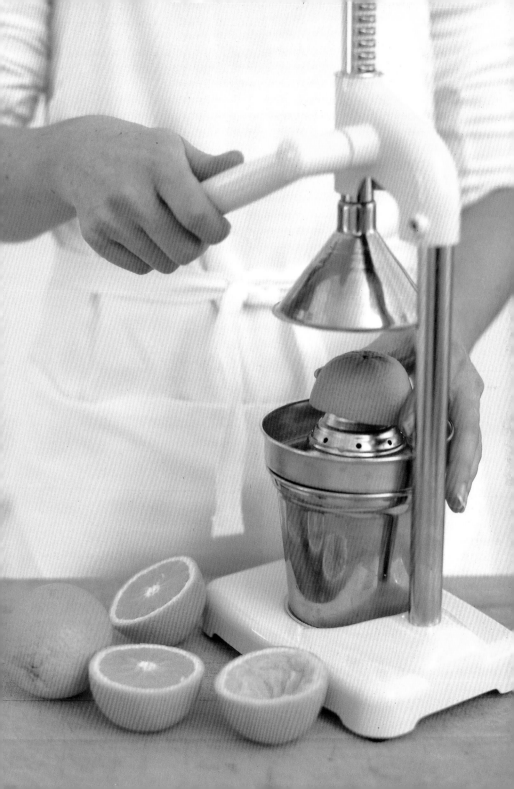

# the detox bonus

There are no two ways about it, we live in a toxic world; whether it's **external pollution**, abusing our bodies with a **poor diet**, or leading too stressful lives, we are all vulnerable.

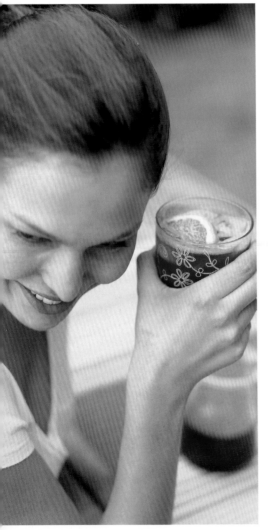

By embarking on this diet, you are not only helping your body shed unwanted pounds, you are also giving your system a chance to detox. By the end of seven days, you could experience restored vitality, more mental clarity, clearer skin and eyes, and a strengthened immune system, which means you'll be looking and feeling healthy in every aspect of your being. By detoxifying your body, you can enjoy these benefits and more.

Practiced for centuries by many cultures around the world—including the Ayurvedic and Chinese medicine systems—detoxification involves resting, cleansing, and nourishing the body from the inside out. By eliminating toxins, then feeding your body with healthy nutrients, detoxifying can help protect you from disease and renew your ability to maintain optimum health.

## how does detoxification work?

Basically, detoxification means cleansing the blood. It does this mainly by removing impurities from the blood in the liver, where toxins are processed for elimination. The body also eliminates toxins through the kidneys, colon, lungs, lymph, and skin. However, when this system is compromised, impurities aren't properly filtered and every cell in the body is adversely affected. Degenerative disease usually springs from either one or a combination of two main conditions: deficiency (not enough nutrients being taken in) or congestion (an excess of toxins from an unhealthy lifestyle).

So cleansing and nourishing the system is vital to the body for overall health. It helps with weight control because it supports two important organs.

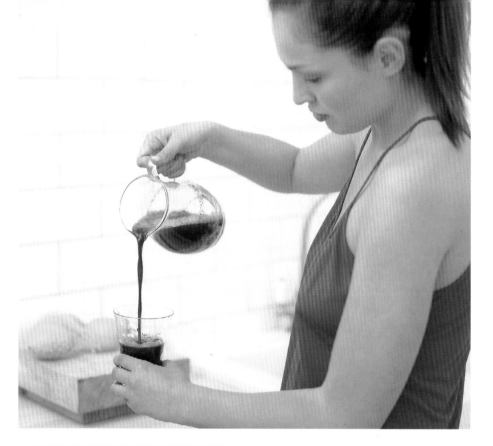

## the liver

Your liver is your body's filter. It has the difficult task of neutralizing many substances that your body either produces as a result of normal metabolism or comes into contact with. If your liver becomes loaded with toxins, it cannot metabolize ingested fats properly, so it dumps them straight back into the bloodstream along with an unhealthy dose of cholesterol. This not only plays havoc with your health, it sabotages weight-loss attempts.

## the colon

Your colon is designed to eliminate body waste along with toxins. The great thing about this diet plan is that it provides the body with masses of enzymes that enable the liver to do its detoxifying job and aid elimination by breaking down and liquefying food in the digestive tract, augmented by an abundance of vitamins and minerals, without which the enzymes couldn't do their good work.

### DID YOU KNOW?

The World Health Organization (WHO) maintains and analyzes cancer mortality (death) rates from 70 countries. WHO research shows that industrialized countries have far more cancers than less developed countries (after adjusting for age and population size). One-half of all the world's cancers occur among people living in industrialized countries, even though this group is only one-fifth of the world's population. From this data, WHO has concluded that at least 80 percent of all cancer is attributable to environmental influences.

# vitamins, minerals, & antioxidants

The work of minerals and vitamins is interrelated and each helps the other to be **absorbed** and **utilized**. So a diet rich in both is essential, particularly when on a weight loss and detoxification plan.

Vitamins are vital to human nutrition and can only be found in living things—that is, plants and animals. Specific combinations of these nutrients, in conjunction with other substances, such as minerals and phytonutrients, make sure that all bodily systems function correctly. If the diet is lacking, then supplementation is essential. This is often the case when a person eats nutritionally depleted food, not enough food, or is putting extra pressure on the body through overwork, during illness or following surgery, or when undergoing high levels of stress.

## fat-soluble vitamins

There are two types of vitamins: fat soluble and water soluble. When you eat foods that contain fat-soluble vitamins, the vitamins are stored in the fat tissues in your body and in your liver, ready to be utilized when your body needs them. Vitamins A, D, E, and K are all fat-soluble vitamins.

## water-soluble vitamins

Water-soluble vitamins are different. When you eat foods that contain water-soluble vitamins, they can't be stored in your body. Instead, they travel through your bloodstream and any excess is expelled in the urine. This group of vitamins includes vitamin C and the big group of B vitamins—$B_1$ (thiamin), $B_2$ (riboflavin), niacin, $B_6$ (pyridoxine), folic acid, $B_{12}$ (cobalamine), biotin, and pantothenic acid.

## minerals

Minerals are nutrients that exist in the body and in food in organic and inorganic combinations. Approximately 17 minerals have been found to be essential to human nutrition. About 4 to 5 percent of human body weight is mineral matter. They are vital to overall health and physical well-being. All tissues and internal fluids of living things contain varying amounts of minerals, and they are also the major constituents of the bones, teeth, soft tissue, muscle, blood, and nerve cells.

There is a clear and important distinction between the terms "mineral" and "trace element." If the body requires more than 100 mg of a mineral each day, the substance is labeled mineral. If the body requires less than 100 mg of a mineral each day, the substance is labeled a trace element.

Minerals are fundamental to maintaining the delicate water balance essential to mental and physical processes. They keep blood and tissue fluids at their correct pH balance and facilitate the passing of other nutrients into the bloodstream. They also help to draw chemical substances in and out of the cells and aid the creation of antibodies. On this diet, care has been taken and advice given to be sure that the full spectrum of vitamins and minerals is part of the daily intake.

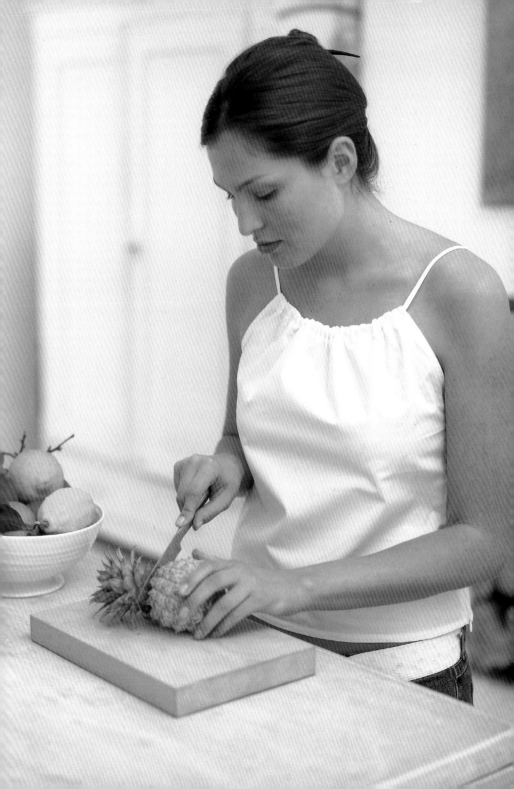

# phytonutrients

Until recently, it was thought that fats, proteins, carbohydrates, vitamins, and minerals were all the **nutrients necessary** for growth and health. Now we know there's **another group** of nutrients necessary for **optimal health**— phytonutrients (from the Greek *phyton*, meaning "plant").

Molecular science is finally confirming that the power-packed nutrients that give fruits and vegetables their many colors also provide a lot of Mother Nature's medicine. While many phytonutrients have been identified, there are probably thousands more that remain undiscovered.

Phytonutrients protect the body and fight disease. They help the cells repair themselves by stimulating the release of protective enzymes or those that rebuild damaged cells. This makes them essential in the fight against cancer. Carcinogens (cancer-causing substances) can enter the body from many sources: tobacco smoke, pollution, pesticides, and chemicals from many manufactured products. Once in the body, these carcinogens can create disease. Phytonutrients inhibit cancer-producing substances, reducing their ability to damage cells. When the repair squad can stay ahead of the damage, degenerative diseases, such as cancer, multiple sclerosis, and arthritis, can't get started. Antioxidant phytonutrients also keep cardiovascular disease in check by blocking the damaging effects of LDL cholesterol on arteries.

## the significance of the Mediterranean diet

This phyto-protective mechanism explains why cultures whose diets are rich in plant foods have the lowest rates of cancer and heart disease. The Mediterranean diet, for example, emphasizes garlic, tomatoes, onions, fruits, whole grains, and olive oil—all of which are rich in phytonutrients.

It's not only what fruits and vegetables contain that make them effective cancer fighters; it's also what they don't contain—saturated and hydrogenated fats, refined sugar and grains, and chemical pollutants frequently found in processed foods.

Whereas a huge amount of information exists about vitamins, phytonutrients are newcomers to the health-food table. The "pill pushers" try to sell them as supplements, although the medical world is still trying to establish their exact role. So if you find the information confusing, follow a few "phyto rules."

* Like other nutrients, phytonutrients operate under the biochemical principle of synergy (1 + 1 = 3). For example, flavonoids and carotenoids have more health-promoting properties when they are eaten together in the same food instead of when they are taken separately in a health supplement. By eating a few florets of broccoli, you're not only getting the beta-carotene you could get in a pill, but you're probably also getting the health benefits of hundreds or thousands of other phytonutrients that don't even have names yet. And, of course, you're getting all the other nutrients, too.

* Each class of phytonutrients affects cellular well-being differently, and the greatest way to take full advantage of the best medicine nature has to offer is to eat a variety of fruits and vegetables.

* Raw vegetables have more nutrients than cooked ones.

# PHYTONUTRIENTS AND THEIR BENEFITS

| PHYTONUTRIENTS | PLANT | BENEFITS |
| --- | --- | --- |
| Allyl sulfide | Garlic and onions | Allicin in these vegetables is a potent antiviral and antibacterial agent. Decreases the risk of stomach and colon cancer, lowers LDL (bad cholesterol), encourages production of the enzyme glutathione S-transferase, which helps eliminate toxins from the body. |
| Lutein | Green leafy vegetables, spinach, turnips, beet tops, collard greens, kale, yellow squashes | This carotene antioxidant protects against degenerative diseases, including macular degeneration. Also protects all body cells from premature aging. |
| Indoles, sulforaphanes | Broccoli, Brussels sprouts, cabbages, other leafy green vegetables | Indoles eliminate toxins, enhance immunity and prevent cancer-causing hormones from attaching themselves to cells. Sulforaphanes remove carcinogens from cells. |
| Isoflavones, such as saponins, phytosterols, genistein | Soy products, cruciferous vegetables, cucumbers, sweet potatoes, tomatoes | Isoflavones are powerful antioxidants that protect against cancer. Genistein prevents the body from taking up dangerous chemical estrogens. Saponins enhance immune functions and help to prevent absorption of cholesterol. Phytosterols lower cholesterol. |
| Lycopene, P-coumaric acid, coumarins | Tomatoes, tomato juice, watermelons, pink grapefruits, papayas, oranges, mangos | From the same family as beta-carotene, lycopene has great antioxidant power and guards against colon and bladder cancer and reduces risk of cardiovascular disease. P-coumaric acid (also found in strawberries and red bell peppers) inhibits the production of cancer-causing nitrosamines in the body. Coumarins reduce inflammation. |
| Limonene, glucarase | Citrus fruits: oranges, tangerines, grapefruits | Limonene enhances immunity and increases production of anticancer enzymes. Glucarase eliminates degenerative chemicals from the body. |
| Alpha-carotene, beta-carotene (carotenoids) | Orange vegetables and fruits: mangos, pumpkins, carrots, sweet potatoes, squashes | Antioxidants with a huge ability to boost immunity and decrease risk of many cancers, degenerative disease, and aging. |
| Polyphenols, flavonoids, anthocyanins | Berries, red grapes, red wine, artichokes, yams | These lower the risk of heart disease, flush out chemicals. Flavonoids fight cell damage from oxidation, strengthen blood vessels and capillaries, improve skin and eyesight |
| Lignan precursors | Flaxseeds | Lignan precursors help prevent cancer and are great sources of omega-3 fatty acids. |

# top 20 fruit & vegetables

This **top 20** is filled with vitamins, minerals, and phytonutrients by the score. **Mix** them up and eat some of **each color** every day.

**1 melons** are highly nutritious, and many melons are natural diuretics, so they are also powerful cleansers and detoxifiers. Because of their high water content, melons are also great for rehydration. Orange melons, such as cantaloupe, are high in beta-carotene. Watermelons have anticoagulant properties and all melons are antiviral and antibacterial.

**2 kiwifruit** are packed with vitamin C and full of fiber. They contain actinidin, an enzyme that is excellent for the immune system, lowering blood pressure, and all-round heart health. They are also known as Chinese gooseberries and are revered in traditional Chinese medicine for their healing effect on stomach and breast cancer.

**3 bananas** are one of the best sources of potassium, an essential mineral for maintaining normal blood pressure and heart function. A banana a day may help to prevent high blood pressure and protect against atherosclerosis. The fiber content helps to prevent cardiovascular disease and the calcium content helps to promote bone health. Bananas contain pectin, a soluble fiber (called a hydrocolloid) that can help normalize movement through the digestive tract and ease constipation. Bananas are an exceptionally rich source of prebiotics that nourish probiotic (friendly) bacteria in the colon. These beneficial bacteria produce vitamins and digestive enzymes that improve our ability to absorb nutrients, plus compounds that protect us against unfriendly microorganisms, and gastrointestinal transit time is lessened, decreasing the risk of colon cancer.

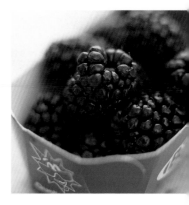

**4 berries** of all kinds do so much for our general health. Fill your freezer with red and purple nutritious berries when fresh are not in season. They are antiviral and antibacterial. Berries of all kinds are fabulous for the bloodstream. Blueberries and black currants help diarrhea and any urinary infection. Raspberries contain natural aspirin and are reputedly good for menstrual cramps. Strawberries are high in pectin, full of lycopene, and benefit the cardiovascular system as a whole.

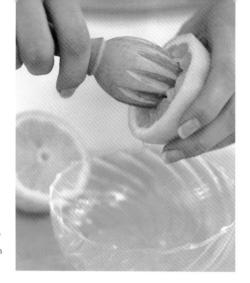

**5** **avocados** are a complete food, packed with essential nutrients. They lower blood cholesterol and contain glutathione, which blocks 30 different carcinogens. The high vitamin E content is excellent for maintaining a healthy skin, healing wounds, and bolstering the immune system. They are also a good source of lecithin, which helps the body digest and metabolize fats.

**6** **cranberries** deodorize urine and prevent bacteria in the bladder, prostate, and kidneys. They have the power to keep the entire urinary tract free from infection because they contain mannose, which is more effective than antibiotics. Cranberries can also help prevent kidney stones and are antiviral and antibiotic. They are sour and so should be combined with sweeter fruit in juices and smoothies.

**7** **citrus fruits,**—collectively oranges, lemons, limes, and grapefruits—contain carotenoids, bioflavonoids, and huge levels of vitamin C that are key in the fight against cancer. They lower blood cholesterol and arterial plaque. Citrus fruits are antiviral, antibacterial, and extremely versatile, because they give a great burst of flavor to any juice or smoothie.

**8** **papayas** are the tops when it comes to aiding digestion, because they contain the enzyme papain, which helps to break down protein. They protect against cancer and replenish lost levels of vitamin C, making them a good choice for smokers.

**9** **apples** are antioxidants, reduce cholesterol, cleanse the digestive system, and boost the immune system. Apples provide an excellent base for many juices, and even a small addition of apple will soften the taste of a stronger vegetable blend. Apples are also full of nutrients that aid in the digestion of fats.

**10** **plums** are full of phenols and are powerful antioxidants. They help increase absorption of iron into the body and are a great source of vitamin C, so are a good immune-boosting choice of fruit. Plums are a good source of vitamin A (in the form of beta-carotene), vitamin $B_2$, dietary fiber, and potassium.

**11** **pineapples** add fantastic flavor to many juices and smoothies. They are anti-inflammatory, antiviral, and antibacterial. They are able to help dissolve blood clots and contain the digestive enzyme bromelain, which is essential in the digestion of protein.

**12** **mangoes** are mighty impressive, self-contained packages of vitamins, minerals, and antioxidants. Mango is a shining star in the beta-carotene realm and is full of potassium. It's the perfect fruit for replenishing energy after a session of heavy physical exercise, such as jogging or working out.

**13** **tomatoes** have got to be the most versatile ingredient known to humans and are fantastic for our health. They lower the risk of cancer and heart disease due to the presence of lycopene, which fights off free radicals. Tomatoes mix well with most other fruits and vegetables.

**14** **broccoli** is a member of the cruciferous (cabbage) family of vegetables. They are loaded with antioxidants and broccoli is pulsating with vitamin C. It is vital to have a regular intake of this vegetable if you want to guard against lung, breast, and colon cancer. On a low-carb program, broccoli is useful because it helps to regulate insulin and blood sugar. It has been reported that it can even deactivate cancer cells.

**15** **cabbages** are a leading cancer fighter. They are full of indoles, can regulate estrogen metabolism, and discourage formation of polyps. Cabbage is definitely best eaten raw and ideally should be included in the diet two or three times a week. As a detoxifier, it is greatly effective and is a great ingredient in juices. The downside? The taste. But if you mix it with more pleasant-tasting fruits and vegetables, the juice can actually be palatable.

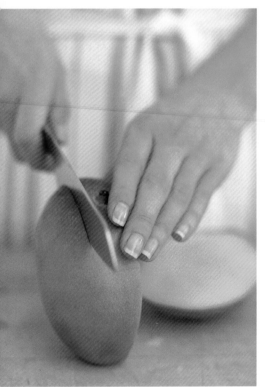

**16** **sweet potatoes** contain unique root storage proteins that have significant antioxidant capacities. Because of their high level of carotenoids, they also help stabilize blood sugar levels and lower insulin resistance. An excellent source of vitamin A (in the form of beta-carotene), a very good source of vitamin C and manganese, and a good source of copper, dietary fiber, vitamin $B_6$, potassium, and iron. Because these nutrients are also anti-inflammatory, they can be helpful in reducing the severity of conditions where inflammation plays a role, such as asthma, rheumatoid arthritis, and osteoarthritis.

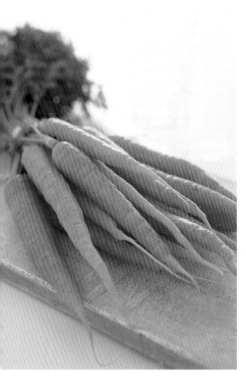

**17** **bell peppers** are rich in vitamin C and have antioxidant properties. They help guard against macular degeneration and respiratory infections. They also help to keep arteries decongested and are said to be effective in helping conditions, such as asthma, bronchitis, and even the common cold. Bell peppers are rich in natural silicones, which help to keep nails, skin, and hair glossy and healthy.

**18** **green leafy vegetables** should be an integral part of the daily diet. Spinach, kale, collard greens, and bok choy are all rich in antioxidants, full of lutein and beta-carotene, and will battle cancer and regulate estrogen. Even if you favor sweeter fruit-based juices, try to have a couple of green juices per week. Your system will thank you for it and glowing health can be yours.

**19** **celery and fennel** are great at cleansing the digestive system of uric acid. They have a high potassium content and are, therefore, great for lowering high blood pressure. If you hold onto excess fluid and experience regular bloating, their diuretic effect is powerful, and if you want to detoxify your body, these should be the basis of the juices you create.

**20** **carrots**, when cooked, rate very highly on the carb scale, less when they are raw, and are too good a juicing ingredient to omit. Used carefully and moderately, carrots are nutritional powerhouses. Their antioxidant capabilities stem from a high beta-carotene content. They fight cancer, protect arteries, battle infections, and boost immunity. They are said to eliminate putrefactive bacteria in the colon and facilitate elimination of intestinal parasites. Carrots are also effective against macular degeneration and blend well with virtually all other ingredients.

# supplements
# & superfoods

Although this is a week-long program based on an abundance of vitamins, minerals, and **health-enhancing** phytonutrients, you will need to take a few things alongside your delicious juices and **smoothies** in order to maintain a healthy balance.

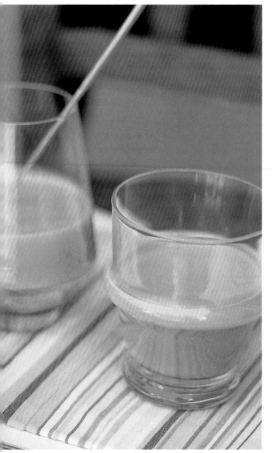

## flax

Flaxseed and flax oil are being rediscovered as true health foods. It is recommended to have a daily tablespoon of flax oil or 2 tablespoons of flaxseed meal. Besides being the best vegetarian source of ALA omega-3, flax oil is a good source of omega-6 or linoleic acid (LA). On this plan, I advise having flaxseed because they contain other nutrients that make eating the whole seed superior to consuming just the extracted oil: a high-quality protein, soluble fiber (the combination of the oil and the fiber makes flaxseed an ideal laxative), vitamins $B_1$, $B_2$, C, E, and carotene, iron, zinc, and trace amounts of potassium, magnesium, phosphorus, and calcium. Flaxseed is high in the phytonutrient lignan. Lignans flush excess estrogen from the body, thereby reducing the incidence of estrogen-linked cancers, such as breast cancer. Besides their antitumor properties, lignans are also antibacterial, antifungal, and antiviral.

Foods high in essential fatty acids, such as flax, increase the body's metabolic rate, helping to burn the excess, unhealthy fats in the body. Eating the right kind of fat gives your body a better chance to store the right amount of fats. This is called thermogenesis, a process in which specialized fat cells throughout the body (called brown fat) click into high gear and burn more fat when activated by essential fatty acids.

**TAKE** two tablespoons crushed flaxseed in one of your daily smoothies.

## psyllium husks

Psyllium is a natural, water-soluble, gel-reducing fiber that is extracted from the husks of blond psyllium seeds (*Plantago ovata*). The bulking effect of psyllium also works to rid the colon of toxic substances, including heavy metals, because it acts almost as a sponge to soak them off the walls of the intestine. This spongy action has a dual advantage; it can decrease hunger when taken with meals. Because psyllium primarily acts by absorbing water and adding more bulk to the stool, it encourages the normal peristaltic (contracting) action of the bowel. Stimulant laxatives, on the other hand, contain chemicals that cause the intestine to increase the secretion of water. They can often create strong contractions of the colon and, if used in excess, can lead to a loss of normal bowel peristalsis and tone. Psyllium also encourages the growth of healthy, "friendly" intestinal bacteria, such as *Lactobacillus acidophilous* and *Bifidobacteria*, which are helpful in regulating bowel movements.

TAKE one teaspoon psyllium husks added to a daily juice or smoothie.

## yogurt

Yogurt disables and kills unwanted bacteria. The probiotics in yogurt with live cultures inhibit the formation of cancer-causing compounds, and they help to detoxify your body by reducing inflammation and encouraging the elimination of intestinal parasites. Yogurt also stimulates the kidneys, thus aiding digestion. If you want a satisfying tasty smoothie, a few tablespoons of plain yogurt with live cultures could be that magic ingredient. Avoid sweetened yogurts, because the sugar content counteracts any beneficial effect—it is antagonistic to the B vitamins that are made from the bacteria naturally found in yogurt.

## fish liver oils

Fish oils (especially cod liver oil) are rich in the EPA and DHA omega-3. These are biologically more potent than the ALA omega-3 in flaxseed. Experimental studies suggest that 3–4 g of ALA per day is equivalent to 0.3 g (300 mg) of EPA per day. EPA and DHA are more rapidly incorporated into plasma and membrane lipids and produce effects more rapidly than does ALA. If you have relatively large reserves

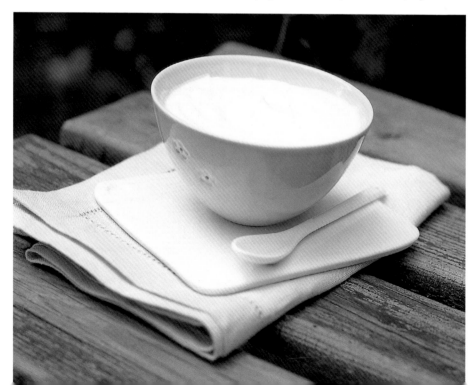

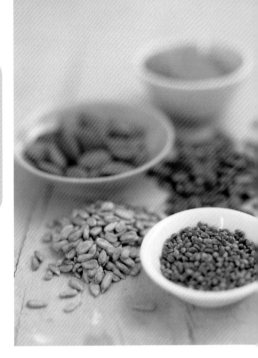

of omega-6 linolenic acid in your body fat (the result of a poor diet high in processed and fried food), these tend to slow down the formation of long-chain omega-3 fats, such as EPA and DHA from ALA.

Incorporating a good-quality fish oil supplement will be beneficial to your diet, because it also provides you with a rare dietary form of vitamin D, which is essential if you have minimum exposure to natural sunlight. And, considering the concerns over high mercury levels in both sea and freshwater fish, refined fish oil supplements may be considered a safer option for your health.

Do check with your physician if you are taking immune system suppressants or cholesterol-reducing medication; certain types cannot be mixed with fish oil supplements.

TAKE the recommended daily dose for adults—usually one capsule (depending on the brand).

## soy

Soy products contain vitamins and minerals in a natural relationship that is complementary to the human body's needs. They are high in isoflavones, which mimic the action of the female sex hormone estrogen (good for menopausal women), reduce insulin levels, decrease arteriosclerosis, and lower levels of LD—bad cholesterol. Soy can help lower the risk of cancer, relieve constipation, regulate blood sugar, and is a major source of protein in vegetarian diets. Try incorporating soy milk, yogurt, ice cream, and tofu into creamy fruit-based smoothies.

## milk thistle

Milk thistle, or silymarin, is believed to have protective effects on the liver and improve its function. It is typically used to treat liver cirrhosis, chronic hepatitis (liver inflammation), and gallbladder disorders. It is an antioxidant, assists in liver cell regeneration, and is used after exposure to chemical and industrial pollutants or adverse effects from excess alcohol or fat consumption. This herb's liver-strengthening properties make it a good supplement to support a juice diet, especially if you think your liver may be overtaxed and is in need of a little extra nurturing.

TAKE the recommended daily dose for adults.

## seeds and nuts

Seeds can be thrown into smoothies for huge boosts of a whole host of vital nutrients. Flaxseed, sesame, pumpkin, and sunflower seeds are rich in protein, the B-complex vitamins, and vitamins A, D, and E, as well as minerals and unsaturated omega-3 fatty acids. Because of their oil contents, they should be kept in the refrigerator or the oils will oxidize, ruining their taste and nutritional value.

Nuts are a concentrated food source. They are full of protein, vitamins, unsaturated omega-3 fatty acids, and minerals, especially selenium, and are an effective anti-oxidant. They reduce levels of bad cholesterol and contain anticancer and heart protective qualities. Add freshly ground nuts to smoothies for extra flavor and nutrition.

## ginger and garlic

Ginger is a fantastic ingredient, long used by Asians for chest congestion, colds, diarrhea, and nausea. It is naturally antibiotic and anti-inflammatory and boosts HDL— good cholesterol. It has also been attributed with antidepressant powers. It strengthens the immune system and can add anything from gentle warmth to fiery heat, depending on how much you throw into the blend.

Garlic is a member of the onion family and has been called the "wonder drug." It is truly one of the world's oldest medicines. Raw garlic is a powerful antibiotic that fights bacteria, parasites, and viruses. Two to three cloves a day lessens the chance of heart attacks and strokes, and garlic contains many anticancer compounds, including allylic sulfides. It boosts immunity and lowers cholesterol and blood pressure. It is at its most powerful when raw,

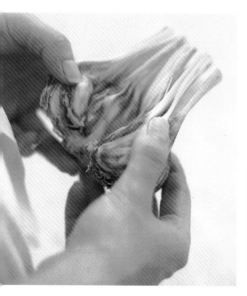

although still potent when cooked. Add a raw clove or two into savory juices for a real health kick.

## brewer's yeast

Brewer's yeast (*Saccharomyces cerevisiae*) is inactive yeast, meaning the yeasts have been killed and have no leavening power. It is the yeast remaining after making beer and is used as a nutrient supplement to increase the intake of the B vitamins. Brewer's yeast is rich in many basic nutrients such as the B vitamins, amino acids, and at least 14 different minerals. The protein content of yeast is responsible for 52 percent of its weight. Because of its B-vitamin content, it is a great physical and mental energy boost between meals. It helps metabolism, is good for eczema, heart disorders, gout, nervousness, and fatigue. Brewer's yeast comes as a powder (the most potent form), in flakes, and in pills. It can be added to drinks, sprinkled over food, or eaten alone. Make sure you use brewer's yeast and not active baker's yeast, because they are totally different in their functions.

Because of its high phosphorus content, it is not recommended for people who have osteoporosis. If you are taking large amounts of yeast, you should make sure to get adequate calcium in the diet. Supplementation of one tablespoon of brewer's yeast a day should be enough. Also avoid brewer's yeast if you have a chronic yeast problem (systemic candidiasis).

TAKE the recommended daily dose for adults, depending on the brand.

### BUYING SUPPLEMENTS

When buying supplements, such as milk thistle and brewer's yeast, buy as good quality as you can afford. Bulk buying may seem like a good idea, but it can be a false economy, because the ingredients may be inferior and lessen the effectiveness of the supplement over time. For maximum freshness, keep all supplements refrigerated in their jars.

# is this the diet for you?

Before you start any diet, you should determine whether it is **appropriate** for you. Consider the various issues raised below before you embark on any **diet plan**.

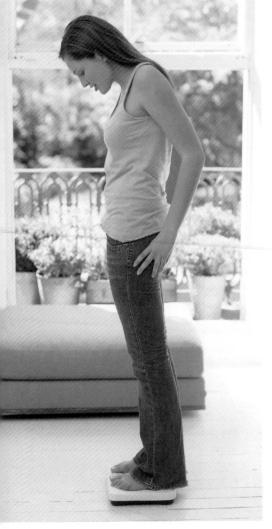

## weighty matters

Are you overweight? If so, how overweight? According to the World Health Organization (WHO), there are more than 1 billion overweight adults globally, at least 300 million of whom are obese. But what is obese? It is easy to over-dramatize your weight predicament and take measures that are overly extreme and unnecessary. Obesity and overweight are words that are often used interchangeably, so let's clarify the difference between obese and overweight. Overweight refers to an excess of body weight, which includes all tissues, such as fat, bone, and muscle, but not necessarily body fat. Obesity means that a person is carrying an excessively high proportion of body fat that could compromise their health.

If you are an athlete or body builder, the chances are you may weigh in at over the desirable weight range for your height (see below) but this is normal because muscle weighs more than fat. You could be a relatively sedentary person who weighs in at the correct weight for your height, but who still carries too high a proportion of body fat for your size. In which case, a good exercise program is vital.

## Body Mass Index (BMI)

The easiest way to determine how severe your weight problem is, apart from simply looking in the mirror or trying to do up your "skinny jeans," is to work out your Body Mass Index (BMI). The BMI is a method of evaluating individual people to see if they are under- or overweight. It involves comparing their weight to their height using the following formula: Multiply your weight in pounds by 700, then divide that figure by your height in inches squared—or use an online calculator. Work out your BMI health by

## RISK OF ASSOCIATED DISEASE ACCORDING TO BMI AND WAIST SIZE

| | BMI 18.5 or less (Underweight) | BMI 18.5–24.9 (Normal) | BMI 25.0–29.9 (Overweight) | BMI 30.0–34.9 (Obese) | BMI 35.0–39.9 (Morbidly obese) | BMI 40 or greater (Extremely obese) |
|---|---|---|---|---|---|---|
| Waist less than or equal to 37 inches in men; 32 inches in women | N/A | N/A | Increased | High risk | Very high risk | Extremely high risk |
| Waist greater than 37 inches in men; 32 inches in women | N/A | N/A | High | Very high risk | Very high risk | Extremely high risk |

using the chart above. A BMI under 18.5 is underweight, between 18.5 and 25 is a healthy weight, and between 25 to 30 is overweight. More than 30 is obese, greater than 35 is morbid obesity, and over 40 extreme obesity.

Now you need to get the tape measure out, because a recent report by the World Health Organization (WHO) suggests that increased risk of chronic and dehabilitating disease is present when the waist measurement of men exceeds 37 inches, and of women, 32 inches. So where do you stand? If your BMI is higher than 30, please check with your physician before embarking on this program.

## detox issues

Although weight loss may be the primary objective and motivation for you choosing this diet, you may need it more than you realize. You might be one of the many people who has learned to live in the "discomfort" zone as a result of a toxic overload from the daily assault of pesticides, additives, antibiotics, hormones, preservatives, and environmental pollutants. Your body may be showing signs of distress and sending you clear messages that all is not well.

Persistent health problems, such as skin disorders, hormonal imbalances, headaches, fatigue, disturbed sleep patterns, and inexplicable pains, particularly under the right shoulder blade, can indicate a toxic liver.

All is probably not well with your colon if you have excessive gas, constipation, or diarrhea, lower back pain, abdominal discomfort, multiple food allergies, or bad breath.

If you have a toxic liver or are experiencing impaired elimination due to a sluggish and toxic colon, along with frequent colds, runny nose, sinus problems, lethargy, mental exhaustion, and premature aging, what you categorically don't have is vibrant health.

## check with your physician

Before you start the diet, it is important to stress that, just like any other dietary program, there are groups of people for whom this diet isn't suitable. If any of the following applies to you, then this may not be your ideal weight-loss plan. In fact, you should check with a qualified medical practitioner before embarking on any new dietary program.

* Pregnant or lactating women
* Diabetics
* Hypoglycemia
* Wilson's disease
* IBS
* Degenerative AIDS
* Presurgery or post-surgery patients
* If you are over 65 or under 18

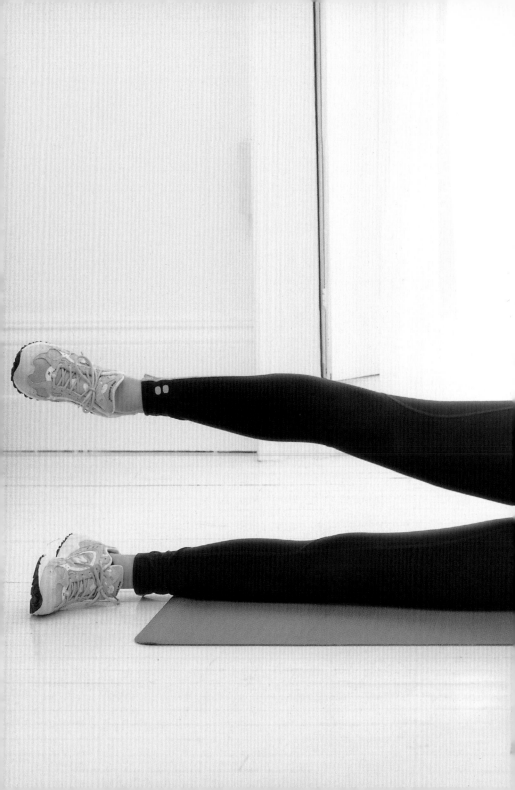

# getting physical

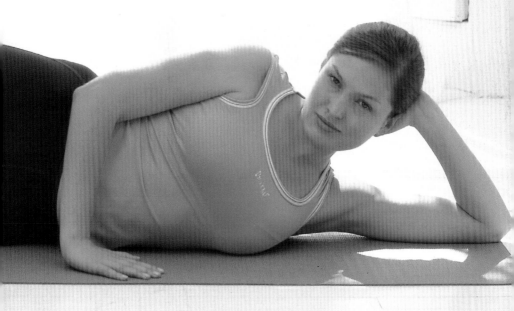

# 10 great exercise ideas

The human body is designed for movement, not slouching in front of the television or bent over a computer. Moving your body is essential if you want to lose pounds and stay fit.

You should aim to exercise for a minimum of 30 minutes a day. However, if the idea of dragging yourself to a local gym and hitting the machines fills you with dread, or the mere mention of the words "aerobics class" brings you out in a rash, don't worry—there are many alternative forms of exercise that may suit you better.

**1** **belly dancing** is wonderful for tightening the muscles of the stomach, waist, and hips and even your thighs. Plus it is amazing for improving posture and relieving back pain, and also perfect for both pre- and postnatal exercise classes.
**Burn around 400 calories an hour.**

**2** **cycling** is something they say you never forget how to do, so why not get on your bike and benefit from a fantastic way to exercise? You can take in some beautiful scenery and get fitter.
**Burn a whopping 600 calories an hour.**

**3** **dancing**, whether gentle ballroom or jigging around your lounge to a few of your favorite tunes, is a fabulous way to say good-bye to those excess pounds.
**Burn between 400 to 700 calories an hour.**

**4** **power walking** is one of the easiest ways to be physically active. You can do it almost anywhere and at any time. Power walking is also inexpensive; all you need is a pair of shoes with sturdy heel support. It is the perfect way to get cardiovascular exercise, not only while on this diet but every day, because it is suitable for most levels of fitness.
**Burn 300 calories in a good one-hour walk.**

**5** **gardening**, if you have a green thumb and a garden to look after, is an enjoyable way to combine a creative hobby and physical activity, but you do need to do the more intensive jobs, such as weeding and pushing a lawn mower, to really burn off those excess pounds.
**Burn around 300 calories per hour.**

**6** **jogging** is cheap, you can do it almost anywhere, and it is a great way to take a little time out and disappear into your own thoughts. It also gets you out and about in the fresh air. Make sure you invest in a decent pair of running shoes to minimize any damaging impact.
**Burn around 300 calories on a 30-minute jog.**

**7** **martial arts** are spiritually, mentally, and physically uplifting exercise experiences that tone every part of your body. If you are the kind of person who can focus and absorb yourself totally in an activity, you will find this very relaxing and invigorating.
**Burn up to 400 calories per hour.**

**8** **jumping rope** will burn serious calories and involves minimal investment—a rope long enough to turn easily. Then all you need is enough space to twirl your rope. Wear comfortable sneakers with a good sole.
**Burn around 300 calories if you skip for 30 minutes.**

**9** **swimming** is a great all-round, no-impact way to exercise your whole body. The more you put in to it, the more you will lose in calorie-burning terms. Wear good-quality goggles to be sure you keep going for longer.
**Burn 200 to 300 calories during a 30-minute swim.**

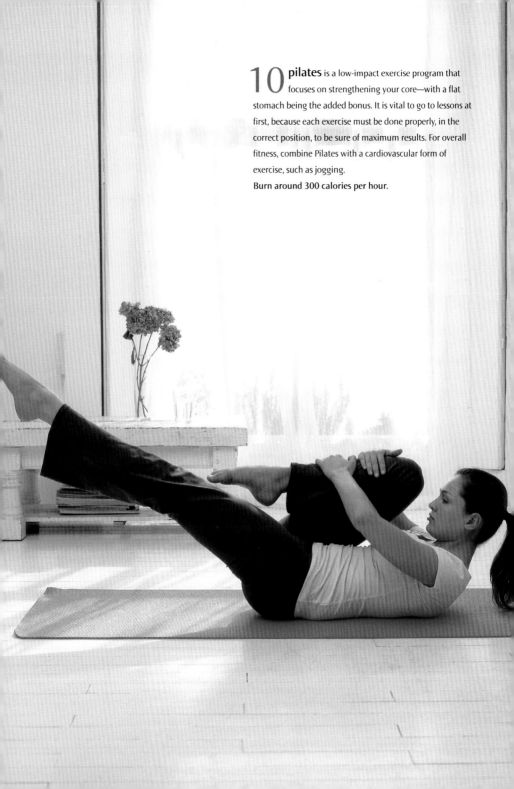

$10$ **pilates** is a low-impact exercise program that focuses on strengthening your core—with a flat stomach being the added bonus. It is vital to go to lessons at first, because each exercise must be done properly, in the correct position, to be sure of maximum results. For overall fitness, combine Pilates with a cardiovascular form of exercise, such as jogging.

**Burn around 300 calories per hour.**

# gentle daily workout

Although training for the marathon or any other form of strenuous exercise isn't a great idea while you are on this diet, you should indulge in regular **physical activity** in order to maximize weight loss. By combining the exercises on the following pages with **30 minutes** of walking each day, you will be well on your way to a healthier, leaner body. As with any exercise program, it is essential that you **warm up** and **cool down** properly.

## warm-up and cooldown
### SIDE REACHES                                        KNEE PULL

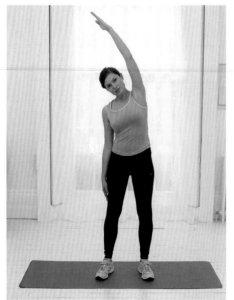 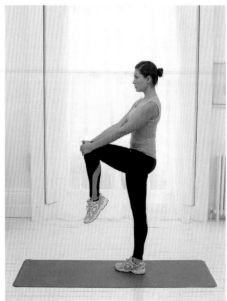

Reach one arm over your head and to the side. Keep your hips steady and your shoulders straight to the side. Hold for 10 seconds and repeat on the other side.

Stand up straight, keeping your head, hips, and feet in a straight line. Pull one knee to your chest, hold for 10 seconds, then repeat with the other leg.

## CALF STRETCH

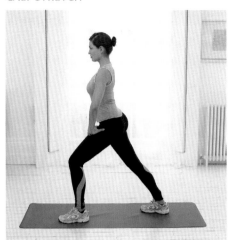

Step forward with one leg and bend your knee. Keep the back leg straight and the foot flat on the floor. Hold for 10 seconds, then repeat with the other leg.

## TRICEP STRETCH

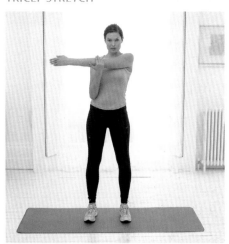

Cross one arm over your chest and pull the elbow closer to your body, using the other hand. Hold for 10 seconds and repeat on the other side.

## THIGH STRETCH

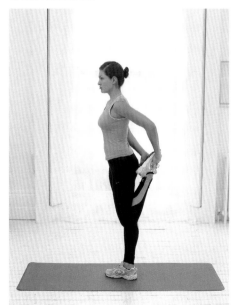

Pull your left foot to your buttocks with your left hand (or both hands). Keep your knee pointing straight to the ground. Hold for 10 seconds. Repeat with your right foot.

## PECTORAL STRETCH

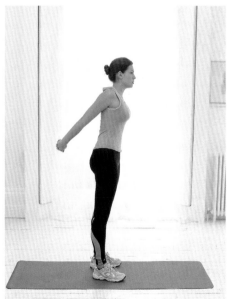

Keeping chest out and chin in, lift your arms behind you until you feel stretch in arms, shoulder, and chest. Hold for 10 seconds.

gentle daily workout    **35**

# upper body
## ARM CIRCLES

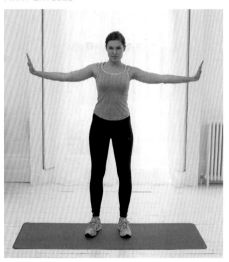

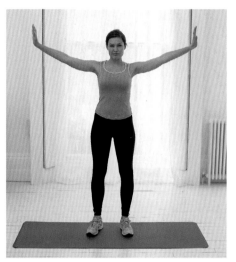

1 Stand up straight with your feet hips' width apart and your arms outstretched to the sides at shoulder height. Move the wrists and palms of your hands in small clockwise circles for the count of 10.

2 Now repeat the movement, counterclockwise, while you count to 10. Repeat the exercise four times.

## CHEST PRESS

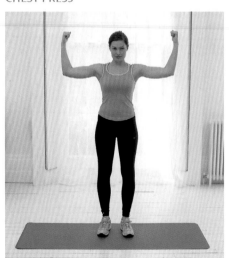

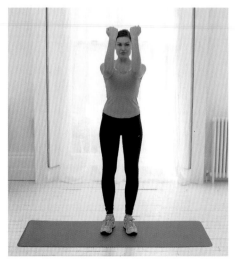

1 Stand up straight, feet hips' width apart. Lift your arms to shoulder height and bend at your elbows.

2 Bring your arms together in front of your body so your forearms press against each other. Return to the starting position and repeat 10 times.

## BICEP CURL

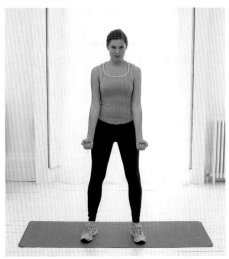 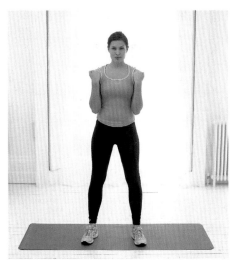

1 Stand up straight with your arms by your sides and fists clenched.

2 Curl your arms toward your shoulders, focusing on the bicep muscles. Lower your arms back to your sides and repeat 10 times.

## GENTLE PUSH-UPS

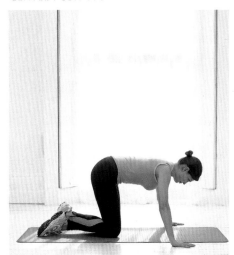 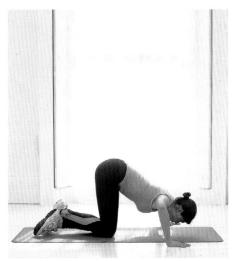

1 Start by kneeling on all fours, with your hands flat on the floor, slightly more than shoulders' width apart.

2 Bend your arms and gently lower yourself down. Return to the starting position and repeat 10 times.

# legs, stomach, and buttocks
## WIDE SQUATS

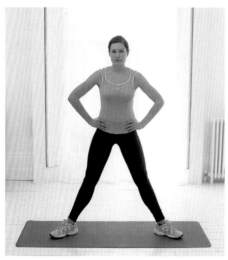

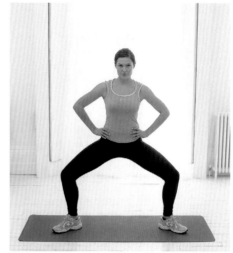

1 Begin by standing with your legs wide apart and hands on your hips.

2 Bend your knees until they are just over your toes, keeping your back straight. Return to the starting position and repeat 10 times.

## CALF RAISES

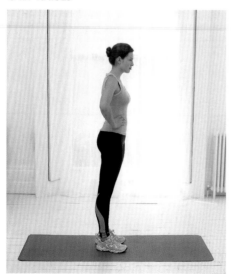

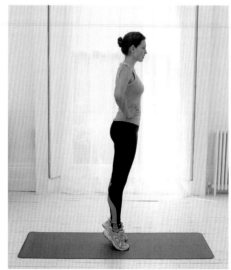

1 Stand up straight with your legs together, your hands on your hips, and your feet flat on the floor.

2 Raise your heels and lift yourself up on to your toes, hold for 1 second, then lower. Repeat 10 times.

## UPPER LEG RAISES

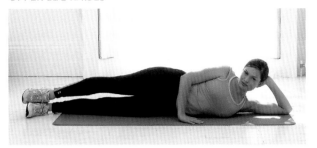

**1** Lie on your side with one leg on top of the other and your hips facing forward. Support your head with your forearm.

**2** Slowly raise the top leg, then lower it back down. Repeat the lift 10 times on the first leg, then 10 times on the other leg.

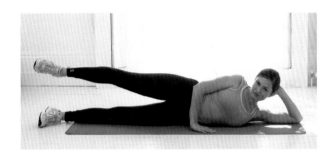

## LOWER LEG RAISES

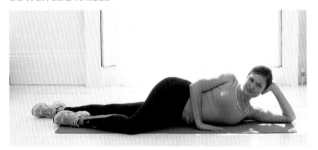

**1** Take up the same starting position as above, then bend the top leg over the bottom leg and rest on the floor, while keeping your hips centered.

**2** Slowly lift the lower leg until it's in line with your body. Hold for 1 second, then lower it. Repeat the lift 10 times on this leg, then 10 times on the other leg.

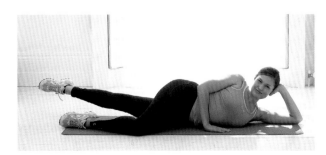

# abs and back
## GENTLE SIT-UPS

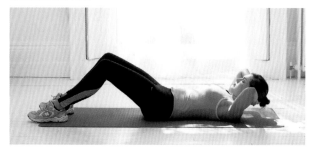

1 Lie on your back with your knees bent and your arms behind your head to support its weight. Contract your stomach muscles, as if trying to push your navel against your spine.

2 Lift your head and shoulders, hold for 1 second, then lower. Repeat 10 times.

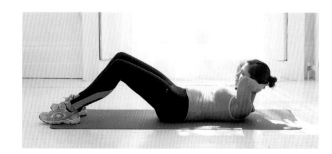

## SIDE CURLS

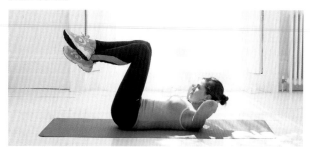

1 Lie on your back with your knees bent at a right angle, your ankles either touching or crossed, and your arms behind your head to support its weight.

2 Lift your head and shoulders and, twisting from your waist, raise your right elbow toward your left knee. Repeat 5 times with the right elbow and 5 times with the left.

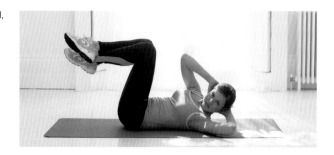

## BACK RAISES

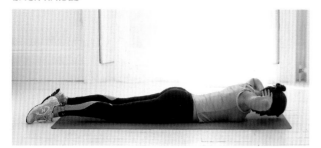

1 Lie on your front with your elbows bent and your hands on the back of your head.

2 Contract your stomach muscles and slowly lift your head, neck, and shoulders off the floor. Lower slowly back down and repeat 10 times.

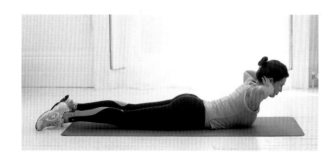

## SIDE-TO-SIDE

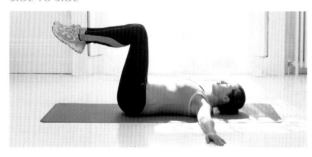

1 Lie on your back, lift your legs and bend your knees so that your shins are parallel to the floor. Stretch your arms out to the sides in line with your shoulders.

2 Contract your stomach muscles, move both your knees to one side, and lower them toward the floor, keeping your shoulders still. Return your legs to the starting position and repeat 5 times on the left side and then 5 times on the right.

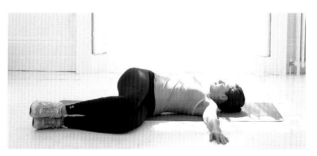

gentle daily workout **41**

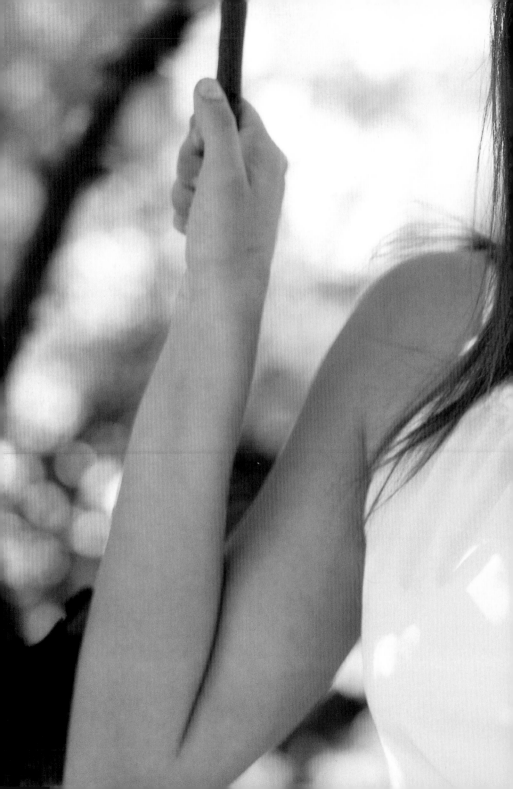

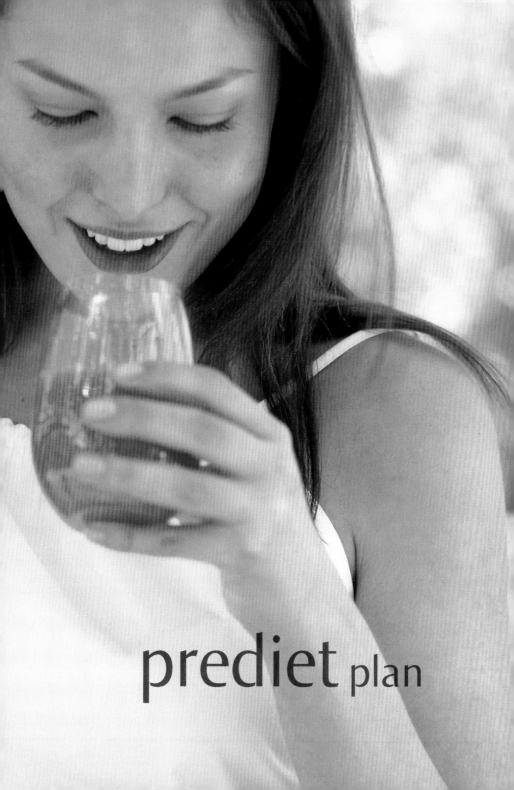

prediet plan

# getting started

Although it might be very tempting to jump straight in and get juicing, please keep in mind that some **preparation** is needed, especially if you smoke, drink caffeine and alcohol, eat junk food, and take medicine at the first sign of discomfort.

Stripping these things from your diet can cause withdrawal symptoms that may cause you difficulty. However, with the correct preparation, this can be minimized.

In order to promote weight loss, this diet will have a detoxifying effect on your body. It will renew and refresh you, but it can cause various side effects as your body rids itself of the toxins that have been keeping you bloated and overweight. As the toxins work their way out from your tissues into the bloodstream, you could experience some of the following common detox symptoms: pimples and rashes, headaches, body odor, bad breath, nausea, runny nose, diarrhea or constipation, flulike symptoms, slight depression, or mood swings. Reactions will differ greatly from person to person, because not everyone is affected equally due to differences in body chemistry. How well we metabolize (break down and get rid of) foreign chemicals depends on our genetic ability and on the extent of the environmental burden of chemicals challenging us.

Even though you may think that you have a healthy diet, toxins aren't just produced by food and drink. Your body will rid itself of any unwanted chemicals, including the chemicals from your own metabolism or that enter your system from the air you breathe, the food and water you consume, substances you put on to your skin or use to treat your hair, or toxins and allergens produced by the germs that inhabit your intestine. However, a few days preparation can minimize any negative side effects, making it easier for you to stick to the plan and maximize your weight loss.

## CUT IT OUT!

For a week before starting the diet, cut out the following:

* Coffee and tea
* Alcohol
* White bread and bread products
* White rice
* Refined sugar
* Salt
* Carbonated drinks
* Juice "drinks" and other soft drinks
* Candy
* Chocolate
* Margarine
* Cookies and cakes
* Potato chips and salted nuts
* Canned fruit and vegetables
* Processed meat products, such as burgers and frankfurters
* Sugary cereals
* Sweet fruit low-fat yogurts
* Ice cream and ice pops
* White pasta
* Prepackaged convenience meals
* Sauces and gravy mixes
* Takeout foods, such as pizza and Chinese

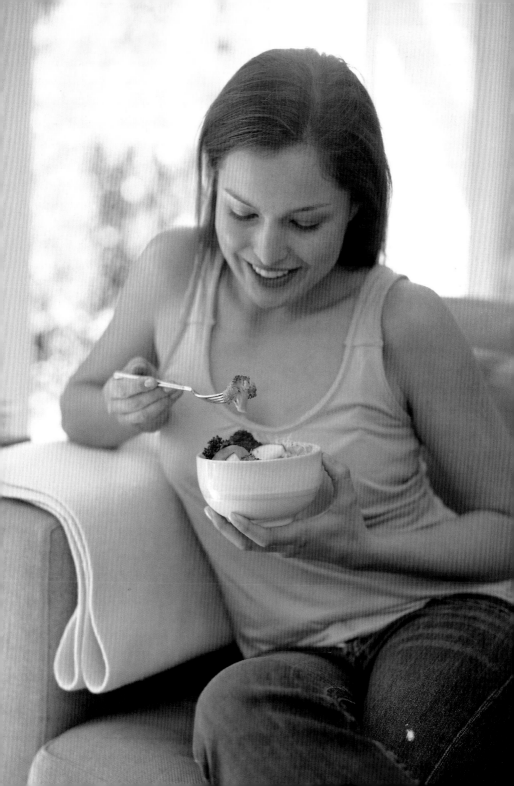

# the baddies

Here are the five big dietary baddies, or as I like to call them, "the **enemies** of your weight and more importantly, your health." Here's why you need to **cut them out** of your diet.

1 **caffeine** I know you are probably reeling in shock—how can you do without your *grande latte*; but sorry, it just has to go. It has a dehydrating effect on your system, which is a disaster if you also don't drink enough water.

You can feel the effects of caffeine in your system within a few minutes of ingesting it, and it stays in your system for four to six hours. While in your body, caffeine affects the following hormones:

* **Adenosine** Caffeine inhibits absorption of adenosine, which calms the body; although caffeine can make you feel alert in the short run, it can cause sleep problems later.
* **Adrenaline** Caffeine injects adrenaline into your system, giving you a temporary boost, but possibly making you fatigued and depressed later on. If you take more caffeine to counteract these effects, you end up spending the day in an agitated state and might find yourself jumpy and edgy by night.
* **Cortisol** Caffeine increase the body's levels of cortisol, the "stress hormone," which can lead to other health consequences, ranging from weight gain and moodiness to heart disease and diabetes.
* **Dopamine** Caffeine increases dopamine levels in your system, acting in a similar way to amphetamines, which can make you feel good after taking it, but after it wears off, you can feel "low." It can also lead to a physical dependence because of dopamine manipulation.

These changes that caffeine makes in your physiology can have negative consequences on your sleep patterns and even your weight. Many experts believe that increased levels of cortisol lead to stronger cravings for fats and carbohydrates, and they cause the body to store fat in the abdomen. (Abdominal fat carries with it greater health risks than other types of fat.)

It is highly addictive, and if you normally consume a lot of coffee, tea, cola drinks, or even chocolate—a not so obvious source—then you will definitely feel the effects if you don't reduce your regular caffeine intake gradually.

Initially, reduce your intake by half, replacing it with a cup of caffeine-free Rooibos tea, herbal teas, or even hot water and lemon. Then after a couple of days, reduce it by half again, and two or three days before you are due to begin the diet (see pages 56–99), eradicate it completely. You will gradually feel your energy rise as your diet improves and your sleep patterns normalize.

2 **refined carbohydrates** In the United States more than 70 percent of the population eats a diet that is high in refined carbohydrates. This is a disaster, because by stripping out the fiber and nutrients from flour and sugar in order to make them look appealingly white, we are making them nutritionally empty.

Food processing removes magnesium, zinc, and chromium from flour and sugar, the three minerals the body needs to metabolize carbohydrates properly. It also drastically reduces vitamins $B_1$, $B_2$, $B_3$, calcium, and iron. So avoid junk foods that are made up of refined flour and sugar, and their equally bad counterparts: processed fats, colorings, flavorings, and preservatives.

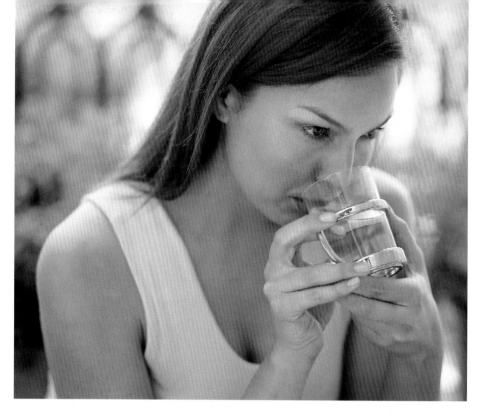

3 **alcohol** Alcohol is probably the most widely abused drug on the planet. Worryingly, the chronic, progressive, and potentially fatal disease alcoholism affects one out of ten people in the Western world. The biggest strain is felt by the liver, which works hard to neutralize the effects of drinking on the body by breaking down the composition of the alcohol. There are many nutrients that can help the liver detoxify alcohol, but, unfortunately, their action is impaired by the alcohol itself, which can interfere with their stores in the body, or prevent the absorption of vital enzymes in the liver that activate these nutrients. For example, the liver will expel all of its folic acid into the bloodstream when alcohol is consumed. This will cause a deficiency that has a knock-on effect. Folic acid is needed to work with vitamin $B_{12}$ to stimulate the formation of red blood cells. Reduce the levels of one of those nutrients and the whole cycle is compromised. Ever wondered why you look so pale with a hangover?

4 **hydrogenated fats** Hydrogenation is one of the processes that can be used to turn liquid oil into solid fat. The final product of this process is called hydrogenated fat. It is used in some cookies, cakes, pastry, margarines, and other processed foods.

During the process of hydrogenation, trans fats may be formed. These are harmful and have no known nutritional benefits. They raise LDL (bad) cholesterol in the blood, which increases the risk of coronary heart disease, and lower HDL (good) cholesterol. Some evidence suggests that the effects of trans fats may be worse than saturated fats.

5 **salt** Although it's been a flavor enhancer and preservative through much of human history, the health effects of salt have aroused suspicion as long ago as ancient China, when excess salt consumption was believed to increase pulse rate. Today, numerous studies have linked high salt intake to a rise in blood pressure. In some people, it could lead to hypertension—pressure higher than 140/90mm Hg, which raises the risk of stroke, heart attack, and kidney damage.

# what to eat

Plenty—of the right stuff, that is. First and foremost are those great **friends of health:** fruit and vegetables, unrefined carbs, and good proteins along with healthy fats and plenty of water.

## fruit and veggies

Allow yourself loads of slow-release carbohydrates from fresh organic fruit, vegetables, and juices in the week leading to the diet. Organic fruits and vegetables contain more vitamins and trace elements and are free from chemical fertilizers and insecticides. Maybe try out a few of the juice recipes.

## carbs

Instead of piling up your plate with fries or pasta, opt for healthy brown rice or a sweet potato in its skin. Have rye bread instead of white or a few healthy oatcake crackers. Experiment with new grains, such as quinoa or millet.

## protein

Boost your body's stores of fat-soluble vitamins by having good-quality protein twice a day. Choose from:

* Fish and shellfish: trout, sardines, mackerel, fresh tuna, cod, bass, sole, herring, canned tuna, haddock, halibut, snapper, swordfish, mussels, squid, oysters, clams, crayfish, lobster, crab, scallops, shrimp, which are all rich in omega-3 fatty acids.
* Poultry and game: organic or free-range chicken, turkey, wild duck, pheasant, quail, rabbit, venison, wild boar.
* Free-range, organic eggs.
* Soy: tofu, tempeh, edamame (soybeans), soy milk, yogurt.

## healthy fats

You will need to have some healthy unsaturated fats, because they contain two fatty acids that are essential to life and that the body cannot produce itself. They are linoleic acid (omega-6) and linolenic acid (omega-3). Out of these two essential fatty acids, your body can make all the other fatty acids it needs. So, do include some healthy fat in your diet and build up your reserves of the fat-soluble vitamins.

Include a little of the following because they are great sources of the right kind of fats:

* Flaxseed oil and flaxseed, hemp oil and hemp seeds, tofu, olive oil, walnuts, sunflower seeds, pumpkin seeds, almonds, avocado, macadamia nuts, olives, tahini.

Even though coconut oil is classed as a saturated fat, it is meant to have health-boosting properties—just don't

---

### PREDIET DIET

Your daily diet should look something like this:

BREAKFAST: Oatmeal with fresh fruit and a dollop of plain yogurt with live and active cultures. OR two poached eggs on rye toast

SNACK: 3 tablespoons sunflower seeds OR one of the juices from the book

LUNCH: Chicken and salad sandwich on rye bread OR tuna salad and an apple

SNACK: A pear OR six to eight Brazil nuts

DINNER: Salmon steak with stir-fried mixed vegetables and brown rice OR turkey breast with steamed vegetables and a small sweet potato

And remember to reduce your caffeine intake.

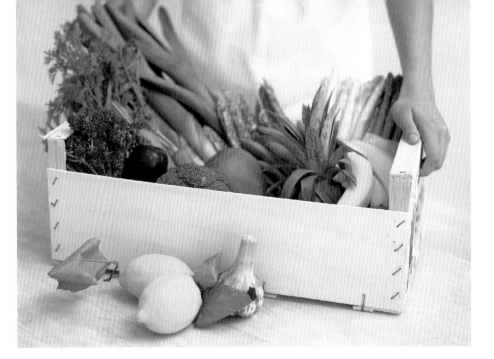

overuse it. Plus, oily fish is also full of omega-3 fatty acids, so don't forget to have at least two to three portions per week.

## water

Drink water, which is essential to start flushing those toxins from your body and keep your system hydrated. Did you know that sometimes when you think that you feel hungry, you are actually thirsty? So try to drink at least eight glasses of water per day.

## the basic rules again

By now you should have a pretty clear idea of what you will have to do, but just to reiterate, here is a basic outline of the rules.

* Prepare for the seven-day juice program by cutting out all caffeine, alcohol, and junk food for at least a week before.
* During this week, eat the majority of your fruit and vegetables in a raw state to be sure of a good level of phytonutrients and fiber.
* Increase your intake of healthy omega-3 fatty acids by eating more oily fish and only using natural unrefined oils in your cooking.

* Eat more high-quality protein, organic if possible.
* Drink at least eight glasses of water per day.
* Incorporate about 30 minutes of aerobic exercise into your daily routine and do the 15-minute gentle stretching and toning session once a day.

## so, are you all fired up?

You should be. You are giving your body a rest from all the bad things you have been eating, and you will be cleansing and nourishing your system. This will help you view food more as vital fuel that allows your body to function at its optimum level. This may be your turning point. You may actually change your attitude from one of "Oh no, I'm on a diet," to a more positive "I am doing this for me, to make myself healthier, fitter, stronger, leaner."

Get excited; pretty soon you are going to be feeling and looking loads better. Think of that boost of self-confidence you are going to experience. All those clothes that have been lurking at the back of your closet, like your skinny jeans, will fit again. So get ready, whatever weight you have to lose, this is only going to work if you are committed to changing your eating and exercise habits for life.

what to eat **49**

# motivational tips

It never ceases to amaze me that people will lavish care and attention on their homes and cars, keep totally up-to-date with the latest high-tech gizmos and gadgets, throw unlimited time and attention into their work, and yet **treat their bodies** with little or **no regard**.

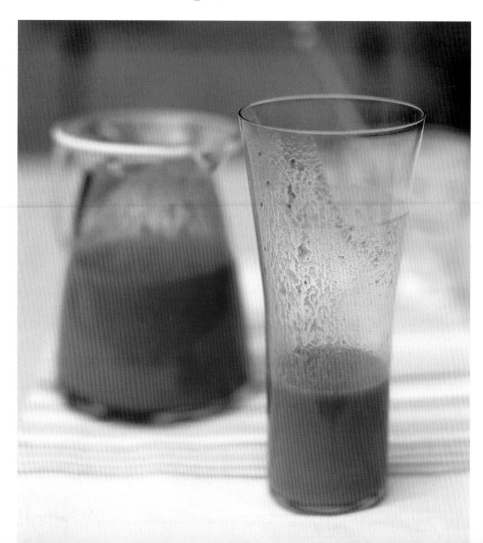

You can buy a new house, cars can be replaced, and you can get yourself a new job, but these things will fade into unimportance if your body starts to let you down. So, maybe it's time to get serious about your health and get yourself into better shape. Don't view the diet as a period of denial; use it as an opportunity to get fitter and feel better.

## the power of five percent

If you are overweight, losing as little as five percent of your body weight may lower your risk of developing the major health problems listed below.

* Type 2 diabetes
* Heart disease and stroke
* Cancer
* Sleep apnea
* Osteoarthritis
* Gallbladder disease
* Fatty liver disease

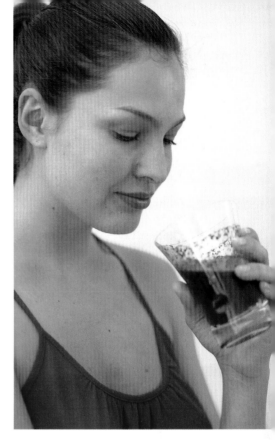

A diet high in sugar can raise insulin levels and develop into diabetes. In 2011, about 26 million people in the United States had type 2 diabetes, a disease that can lead to blindness and amputations. Additives can stimulate the production of hormones that can encourage the growth of certain cancer cells. Junk food also contains unhealthy fats that can raise cholesterol levels and lead to heart disease. According to the World Health Organization (WHO), more than 85 percent of major diseases are caused by what we put into our mouths.

## germ warfare

Your immune system is designed to defend you against millions of bacteria, microbes, viruses, toxins, and parasites that are continually trying to invade your body. This diet will help keep you well on a daily basis, because all the juices and smoothies are bursting with immune-boosting nutrients, such as vitamins A and C. Plus, they also contain all the minerals and phytonutrients necessary to enable successful absorption and utilization of these vitamins. As a result, you won't be so prone to minor ailments, such as colds and flu, and you will be strengthening your resistance to more serious conditions.

## put the spring back in your step

Caffeine is the most widely used drug in the world, and it's no coincidence that its use has increased alongside longer working hours. Along with regular sugar consumption, it is the stimulant of choice for many people who would vehemently deny that they had any form of addiction. Yet both those substances play havoc with energy levels and cause mood swings and fatigue. Throw alcohol into the equation and you will have a body that is suffering from extreme stress; from a health perspective this is a time bomb waiting to explode.

Even though you may find this hard to believe, your energy levels will soar after a few days on the diet, especially if you have been diligent about following the advised preparation plan (pages 44–49) and minimized the withdrawal symptoms. You will be more productive, sleep better, and feel refreshed.

# how to juice

**If you are going to incorporate healthy juices and smoothies into your life, the first step is to get yourself equipped with the proper appliances.**

My best advice is to spend as much as you can afford on reputable brand-name, good-quality machines. Cheaper ones may seem a bargain, but they seem not to be able to stand regular use, and often the cheaper the juicer, the lower quality the juice. Shop around, look online for special offers, but get the best machines you can afford.

## HELPFUL JUICING HINTS

* Use fresh, firm fruits and vegetables for maximum nutrient content.
* Wash all fruits and vegetables thoroughly to remove any dirt or chemicals.
* Remove all stems and large pits.
* Do not force fruits and vegetables through the juicer. Pass them through slowly and steadily, using the pusher provided; never use knives or other metal kitchen implements.
* Do not cut fruits and vegetables too small—cut to a size that fits comfortably into the chute.
* Alternate soft fruits and harder fruits and vegetables; this will help push the softer fruits through.
* When juicing leafy vegetables, roll into a ball and push them through, followed by harder fruit or vegetables.
* Don't try to juice bananas, avocados, or really overripe fruit—they will clog up the juicer. Use them in smoothies.
* Never juice rhubarb, eggplant, coconut, or leeks.

You may already have a citrus press, which is fine for extracting juice from citrus fruit, but in all honesty, it is better to use a proper juicer because you will benefit from the nutrients held in the pith and seeds.

## blender

Look for a sturdy, well-made blender that has a variety of speeds, because you will need to be able to crush ice and blend frozen fruit. Handheld immersion blenders are not really designed to do this and could be messy unless you have a deep container. The liquid will fly everywhere.

## juicers

There are two main types of juicer: centrifugal and masticating. Whichever you choose, the key point to note is that the drier the pulp, the more effective the juicer.

* **Centrifugal** This is the most widely used and affordable juicer. The fruits and vegetables are fed into a rapidly spinning grater and the juice and pulp are separated, but a smaller amount of juice is produced than by a masticating or pulverizing juicer.
* **Masticating** The larger, more expensive juicers operate by masticating or pulverizing the fruit and vegetables. These are pushed through a wire mesh; the action is powerful and produces a high level of juice with dry pulp. The juice is more nutrient-dense, because not only is there more of it, the juice hasn't been extracted via a spinning metal blade that produces heat, which, in turn, kills those vital enzymes.

## cleaning chores

The most aggravating aspect of juicing is cleaning the machine. It has to be done as soon as you have finished juicing, and it has to be thorough, because any residue will encourage bacterial growth. So look out for a machine that dismantles easily.

Most machines come with a special brush to clean the mesh or grater. I have found wire-cleaning pads excellent for the job. Soaking in warm soapy water can also make the task a little easier. If the plastic parts of the machine become stained, use a mixture of one part white vinegar to two parts water to remove the discoloration.

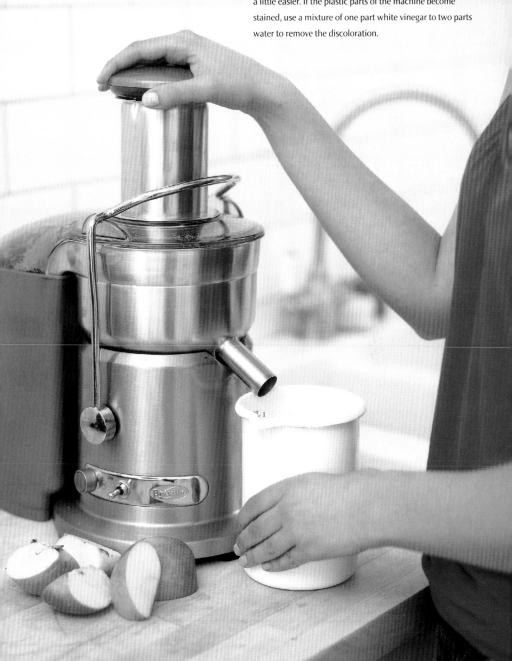

# monitoring weight loss

There are definitely two schools of thought on how to do this: either you go for the daily **weighing** or the once a week weigh-in.

This is an entirely individual issue. If you are the type of person who needs that daily date with your bathroom scale, then by all means do it. If you prefer the "surprise at the end of the week" approach, then this is fine, too. Hhatever your preferred method of keeping track of your progress, you should have a tight-fitting pair of pants or other item of clothing that is a little too close for comfort, and try it on at the beginning and end of the seven days. On a more long-term basis, if you are exercising regularly and increasing your muscle-to-fat ratio, you may even end up weighing slightly more, because muscle tissue is heavier, but your shape will be trimmer.

## dietary demons

One of the most difficult things to deal with when you are trying to stick to a diet is the friend or relative who tries to lure you off course. You know the ones; they usually arrive with a little treat and try to persuade you that one little deviation won't matter. It will. Don't be bullied into breaking your resolve. Politely decline and say that you are relying on them for support. If you are visiting, take a juice or smoothie with you. Even better, if those friends could do with losing a few pounds, try to get them to join you.

## snack attacks

Although you should feel satisfied on this diet, you could undermine your efforts easily by hitting the cookie jar in a moment of weakness. It really is better to clear out anything vaguely tempting from the refrigerator and pantry. If you have a family and this isn't possible, then you will have to be careful, particularly at times that you normally seek a little comfort food.

One woman who couldn't stop herself from snacking on her kids' leftovers used to douse the plates in dish-washing liquid the minute the kids left the table. A little extreme, but unless you like cold fries and chicken nuggets with a side order of soap, it might be an effective way to keep temptation at bay.

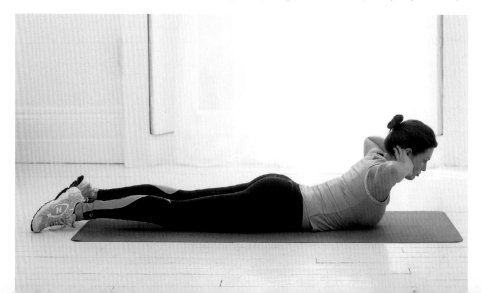

# shopping list

Careful planning is essential when embarking on this diet to be sure you have all of the **ingredients necessary** to prepare the juices and won't be tempted to cheat.

If you have a large enough refrigerator and freezer, one big shopping trip will be enough, but if your space is limited, then you may find you need to shop twice, which is good from the freshness perspective. As mentioned earlier, freezing juices works well, but it may not be practical to make all 35 drinks at one time. It might be more practical for you to make the majority of your juices and smoothies the night before.

## FROM THE HEALTH FOOD STORE

Dried apricots

Brewer's yeast—B-complex

Flaxseed

Milk thistle (silymarin) supplements

Probiotics

Psyllium husks

Sunflower seeds/pumpkin seeds

Variety of unsalted nuts

## FROM THE CHILLED FRESH FOOD SECTION

Cranberry juice

Plain yogurt with live cultures

Tomato juice

## FRESH HERBS

Basil

Fresh chiles

Cilantro

Mint

## FRUITS

Apples

Avocado

Banana

Blackberries, frozen or fresh

Blueberries, frozen or fresh

Cherries

Clementines

Grapefruit

Grapes

Kiwifruit

Lemons

Limes

Melon

Mango

Oranges

Papaya

Passion fruit

Pears

Pineapple

Plums

Raspberries, frozen or fresh

Strawberries

## VEGETABLES

Beet

Bell peppers, red, green, yellow, orange

Broccoli

Carrots

Celery

Cucumber

Fennel

Fresh ginger root

Onion

Red cabbage

Spinach

Scallions

Sweet potato

Tomatoes

Watercress

## DRIED HERBS AND SPICES

Camomile

Cloves

Dandelion

Fennel seeds

Star anise

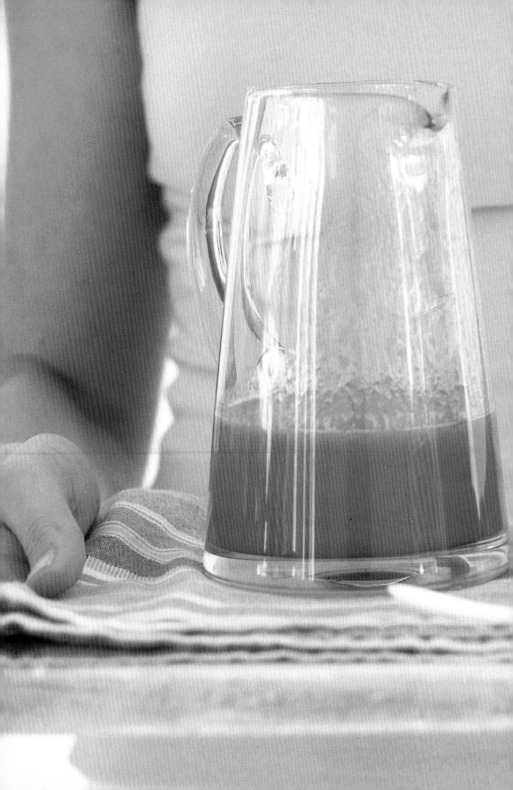

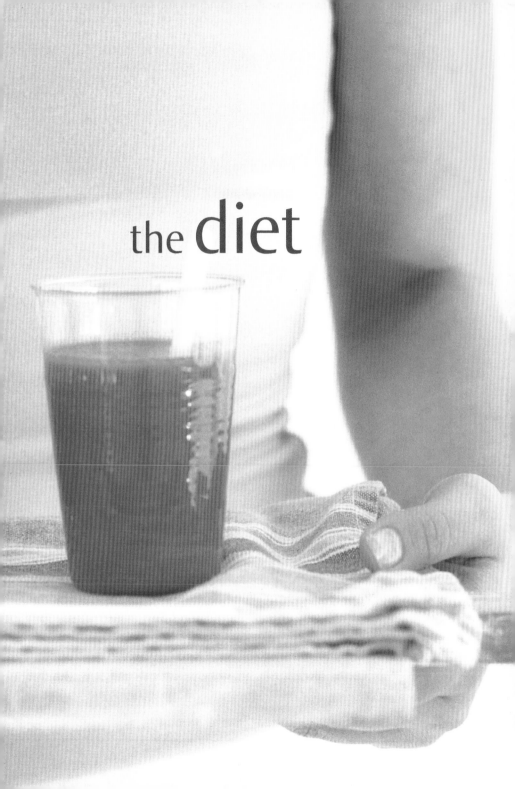

the diet

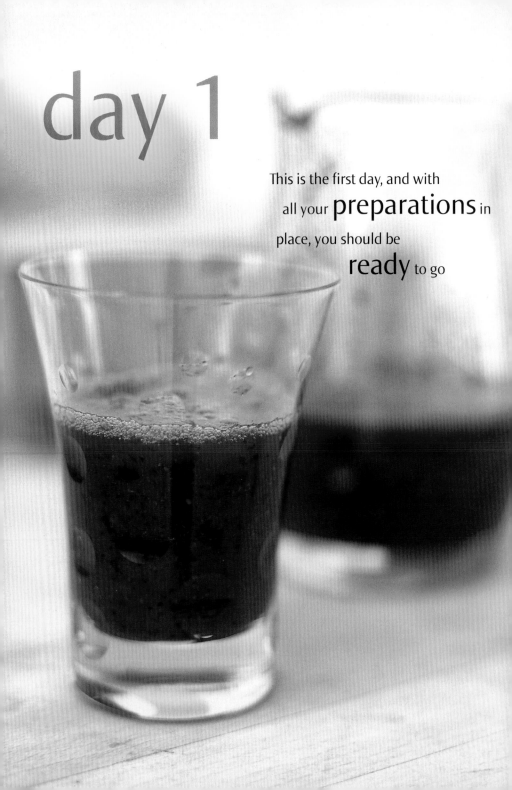

# day 1

This is the first day, and with all your **preparations** in place, you should be **ready** to go

OK, day one is here. Let your juicer and blender take center stage in the kitchen. If you have followed the advice for the preparation week, you should be totally in the zone and already feeling a little lighter and a lot healthier. Good luck.

## ◄ flat belly berry

Apples are excellent for cleansing the system and, along with blueberries and cranberries, they are packed full of vitamins C and E, and the minerals calcium, magnesium, and phosphorus.

3 apples
²/₃ cup unsweetened cranberry juice
1 cup fresh or frozen blueberries
1 tablespoon psyllium husk powder

Juice the apples, and then process the apple juice in a blender with the cranberry juice, blueberries, and psyllium husk powder.

Makes 10 fl oz or 1 large glass
Vitamin C 70 mg • Magnesium 25 mg • Calories 270

## on today's menu

### start the day
Lemon and Ginger Infusion (page 62)

### and then on to
Flat Belly Berry (page 59)
Spicy Pear (page 60)
Lean Green (page 60)
Chile Orange (page 62)
Big Red (page 62)

### and wind down with
Any herbal tea or infusion of your choice
2 teaspoons flaxseed

### snack attack
3 tablespoons sunflower seeds plus 1 apple

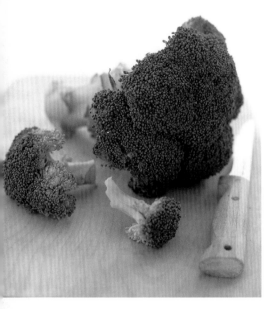

## spicy pear▶

Pears are a gentle laxative, while celery acts as a diuretic and ginger root promotes good digestion, making this a great juice for keeping your system balanced.

1 small pear
2 celery sticks
1 inch piece of fresh ginger root

Juice all the ingredients together and either serve over ice or process in a blender with a couple of ice cubes for a smoother, creamier drink.

Makes 10 fl oz or 1 large glass
Vitamin C 30 mg • Calcium 110 mg • Calories 75

## lean green

Refreshing, green, and healthy, this sweet and savory juice is bursting with goodness.

1¼ cups pineapple chunks
1½ cups broccoli pieces
1 cup cucumber chunks
1 kiwifruit

Juice the pineapple and broccoli, then blend with the cucumber and kiwifruit along with a couple of ice cubes.

Makes 10 fl oz or 1 large glass
Vitamin C 160 mg • Calcium 128 mg • Iron 2.7 mg • Calories 161

### TOP TIP

Instead of drinking your juices and smoothies quickly, take time to actually taste and enjoy the flavors. Let the juice rest in your mouth for a while, because this will stimulate the production of the salivary digestive enzyme amylase.

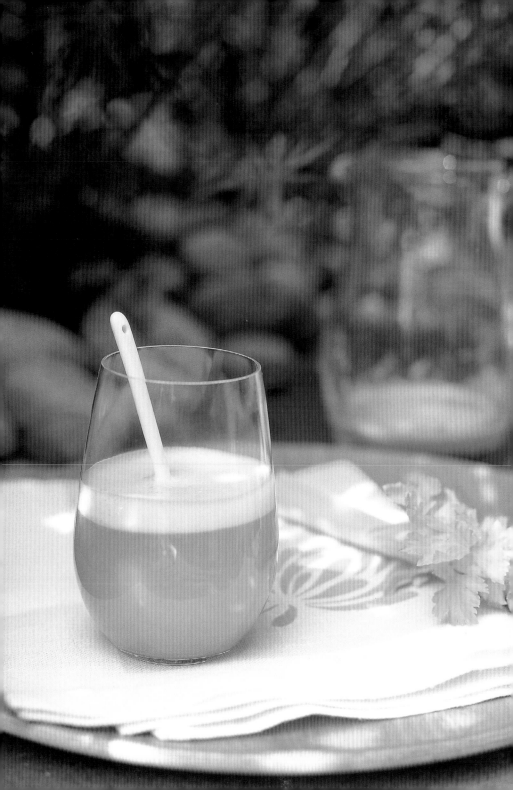

## chile orange

This juice is full of vitamin C, and the enzymes in the pineapple are great at dissolving the mucus that can accumulate in your system if you have a buildup of toxins. The chile not only gives this juice a kick, but is rich in carotenoids.

4 carrots
1 1/2 cups pineapple chunks
1/2 lime, peeled
1/2 small chile, seeded
1 tablespoon chopped cilantro leaves

Juice the carrots, pineapple, and lime, then throw into a blender with the chile, cilantro, and a couple of ice cubes.

Makes 7 fl oz or 1 small glass
Vitamin C 72 mg • Selenium 4 mcg • Calories 240

## big red

This juice is full of phytonutrients, including lycopene, which has been proven to have anticancer properties.

1 1/4 cups hulled strawberries (about 8 oz)
4 tomatoes
a few basil leaves

Juice all the ingredients together and serve over ice cubes.

Makes 14 fl oz or 1 very large glass
Vitamin C 222 mg • Calcium 60 mg • Magnesium 48 mg
• Calories 122

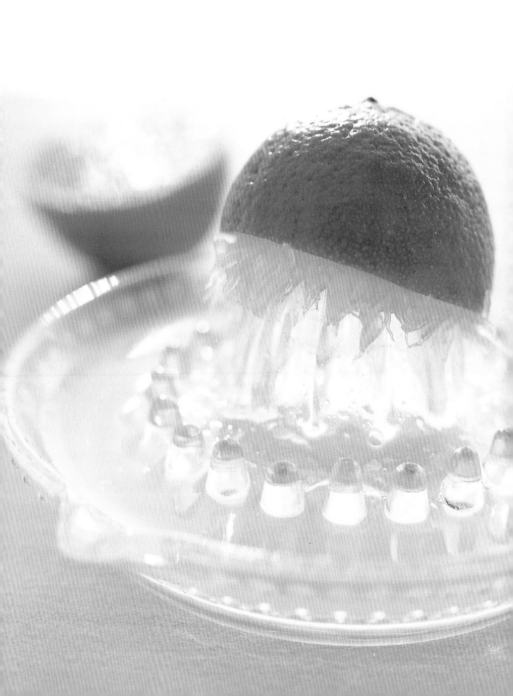

# day 2

If you feel the need **to weigh** yourself, go ahead if you think it will keep you motivated

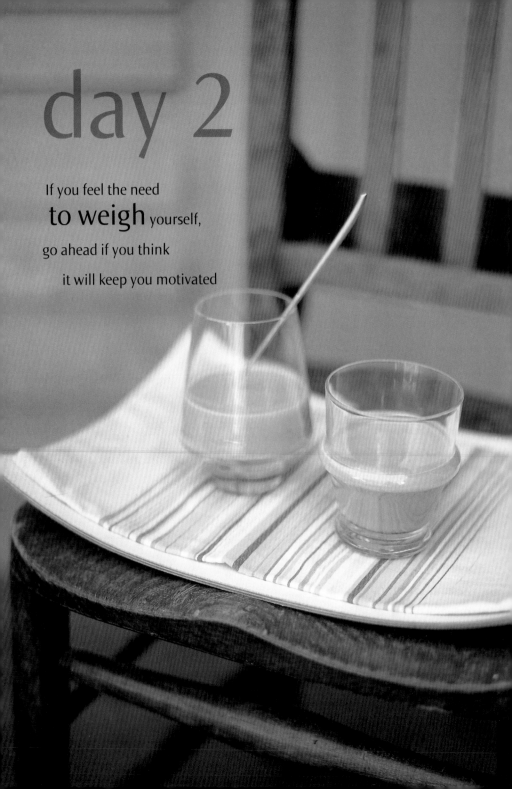

How are you feeling today? Probably a lot better than you thought you might. Get ready for your first smoothie of the day, which is really delicious and very satisfying. You will notice that you feel less bloated than usual, because your body will already be expelling excess fluids from your tissues.

## ◀ orange super smoothie

This nourishing smoothie is rich in iron, calcium, and potassium and high in beta-carotene. Add a handful of sunflower seeds to rev up the omega-3 levels. It will appeal to all the family, especially children, so maybe make extra as a perfect breakfast drink.

1 large carrot
1 orange
1 small banana
1 fresh or dried apricot
variation: swap banana for ¹/₂ small avocado

Juice the carrot and orange. Process the juice in a blender with the banana (or avocado, if that's what you're using), apricot, and a couple of ice cubes.

Makes 7 fl oz or 1 small glass
Vitamin A 44,570 iu • Vitamin C 101 mg
• Potassium 1,475 mg • Iron 2.5 mg • Calories 204

## on today's menu

### start the day
Fennel Infusion (page 69)

### and then on to
Orange Super Smoothie (page 65)
Time Bomb (page 66)
Ruby Smoothie (page 66)
Spicy Lemonade (page 69)
Invigor8 (page 69)

### and wind down with
Any herbal tea or infusion of your choice
2 teaspoons flaxseed

### snack attack
2 tablespoons pumpkin seeds plus 1 pear

## ruby smoothie

This highly nutritious and satisfying smoothie is high in vitamin C, and the combination of the pectin in the apple and probiotics in the yogurt makes it a great choice for the digestive tract.

2 oranges
1 apple
$^2/_3$ cup raspberries, fresh or frozen
$^1/_2$ cup hulled strawberries, fresh or frozen
$^2/_3$ cup plain yogurt with live cultures

Juice the oranges and apple, then process the juice in a blender with the raspberries, strawberries, and yogurt. Serve immediately.

Makes 14 fl oz or 1 very large glass
Vitamin C 145 mg • Vitamin E 1.81 mg • Calcium 407 mg
• Iron 2 mg • Zinc 1.65 mg • Calories 283

## time bomb ▶

All three ingredients in this bright green juice are high in magnesium and vitamin C, which is essential for healthy functioning of the adrenal glands and the liver. If you are going through a prolonged period of stress, your body may be lacking these two vital nutrients, because they are easily depleted when the going gets tough.

5 cups spinach
$^1/_4$ head of broccoli
2 medium tomatoes

Wash all three ingredients and juice. Serve in a glass with a stick of celery, if desired.

Makes 7 fl oz or 1 small glass
Vitamin A 14,234 iu • Vitamin C 202 mg
• Magnesium 171 mg • Calories 120

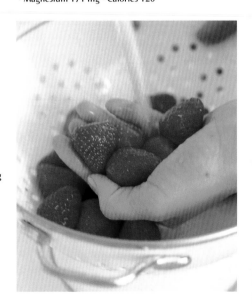

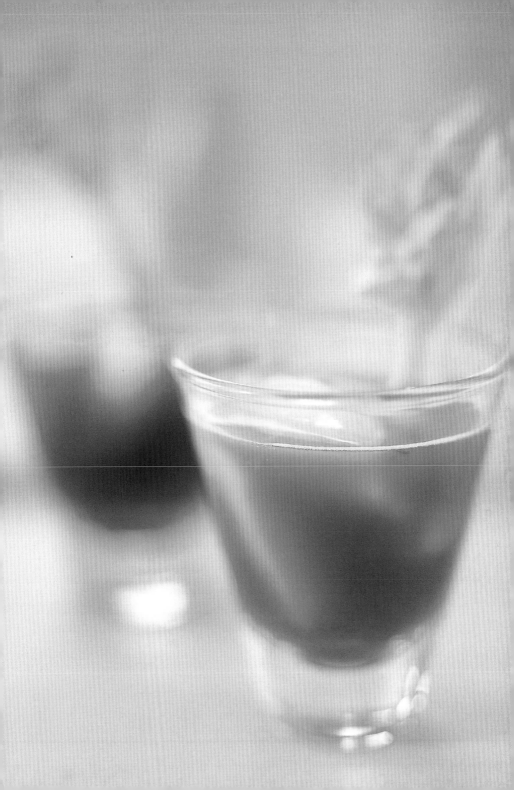

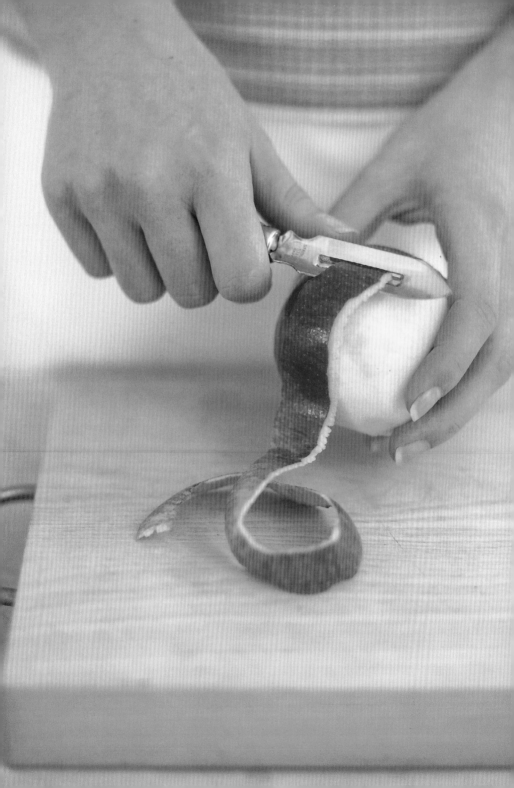

## spicy lemonade

This is great diluted with a little hot (not boiling) water and served as a warm drink. A little cinnamon sprinkled over the top tastes great, and if you like your drinks sour, add an extra squeeze of lemon.

3 apples
$^1/_2$ lemon, peeled
1 yellow bell pepper, seeded
1 inch cube fresh ginger root

Juice all the ingredients together and serve over ice cubes.

Makes 8 fl oz or 1 small glass
Vitamin C 190 mg • Calcium 37 mg • Magnesium 52 mg
• Calories 247

---

### FEEL-GOOD FACTOR

Give yourself a "closet makeover"—if you haven't worn it for a year, give it to a friend or charity. This will free up closet space, help others, and create room for all those fabulous new clothes you'll be able to wear when you are lighter. So go on, chuck it all on the bed, formulate a few new combinations, and be ruthless with yourself. The closet is no place for nostalgia; you just end up looking dated.

---

### LITTLE HOTTY
#### FENNEL INFUSION

Take a tablespoon of fennel seeds and place in a cafetiere or teapot. Cover with boiling water and let steep for 3–5 minutes. Drink freely throughout the day. Fennel is a natural diuretic.

## invigor8

This is an absolutely great juice—a low-calorie, virtually fat-free burst of goodness that will enliven your whole body and help lower blood pressure, aid digestion, boost the immune system, and eliminate toxins. If your stress levels have risen to unhealthy heights, this is the best all-round juice you could have, particularly if you are prone to migraines and nausea.

2 medium oranges
$^1/_2$ lemon
2 beets
$3^1/_2$ cups spinach
$2^1/_2$ celery sticks
2 small carrots
$^1/_2$ inch cube fresh ginger root

Peel the oranges and lemon, then juice along with the rest of the ingredients. Serve in two large glasses.

Makes 20 fl oz or 2 large glasses
Vitamin C 510 mg • Vitamin A 34,736 iu
• Magnesium 164 mg • Folic acid 310 mcg
• Calories 286

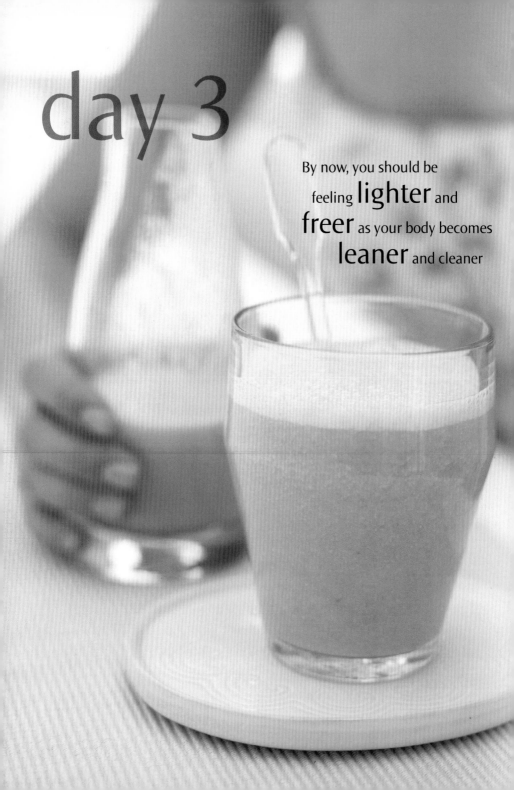

# day 3

By now, you should be feeling **lighter** and **freer** as your body becomes **leaner** and cleaner

You've had two days on the diet. A bit daunted by the prospect of another five days and being faced with temptation? Don't worry, it's much easier than you think. If you take a little time in the morning to make the day's juices and store them in airtight thermoses, they will be ready for you to enjoy when your willpower weakens.

## ◄ banana calmer

When you are really up against it and want a quick breakfast or lunch, this smoothie is high in a wide range of nutrients and is quick to prepare.

1 small banana
1 cup freshly squeezed orange juice
3 tablespoons sunflower seeds

Throw all the ingredients into a blender with a couple of ice cubes and process. Serve in a large glass and decorate with some strawberries, if desired.

Makes 10 fl oz or 1 large glass
Vitamin C 220 mg • Magnesium 113 mg
• Tryptophan 85 mg • Calories 340

## on today's menu

### start the day
Dandelion and Mint Infusion (page 75)

### and then on to
Banana Calmer (page 71)
Deep Breath (page 72)
Hi Tension (page 72)
Power Pack (page 75)
Eye Opener (page 75)

### and wind down with
Any herbal tea or infusion of your choice
2 teaspoons flaxseed

### snack attack
3 tablespoons walnut pieces plus 1 orange

# hi tension

Pineapple contains bromelain, an enzyme that aids digestion and is similar to stomach acid. It is also meant to be highly effective at dissolving blood clots. The only downside is that it is not particularly kind to tooth enamel and is better if drunk diluted. Celery is the perfect accompaniment, because it also aids digestion and lowers blood pressure. This juice is good for reenergizing, detoxifying the liver, and replenishing lost fluids.

1 cup pineapple chunks
3 celery sticks
$^1/_2$ lemon, peeled

Juice all the ingredients. Serve over ice in a tall glass with some sprigs of fresh mint or fennel, if desired.

Makes 7 fl oz or 1 small glass
Vitamin C 33 mg • Magnesium 41 mg • Calories 101

# deep breath ▶

If you are stressed you will often find that your digestion and circulation are affected, which will leave you feeling fatigued and lacking in energy. Red bell peppers are excellent at reducing blood pressure and papaya is renowned for its digestive properties.

1 large tomato
1 red bell pepper, seeded
$^1/_2$ papaya, peeled and seeded

Juice all the ingredients. Blend the juice with a couple of ice cubes in a blender.

Makes 7 fl oz or 1 small glass
Vitamin C 315 mg • Vitamin A 10,851 iu
• Magnesium 51 mg • Calories 124

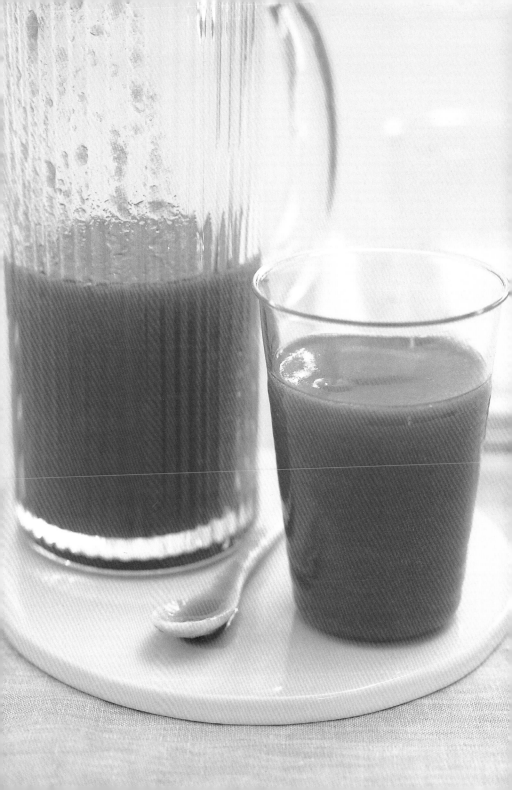

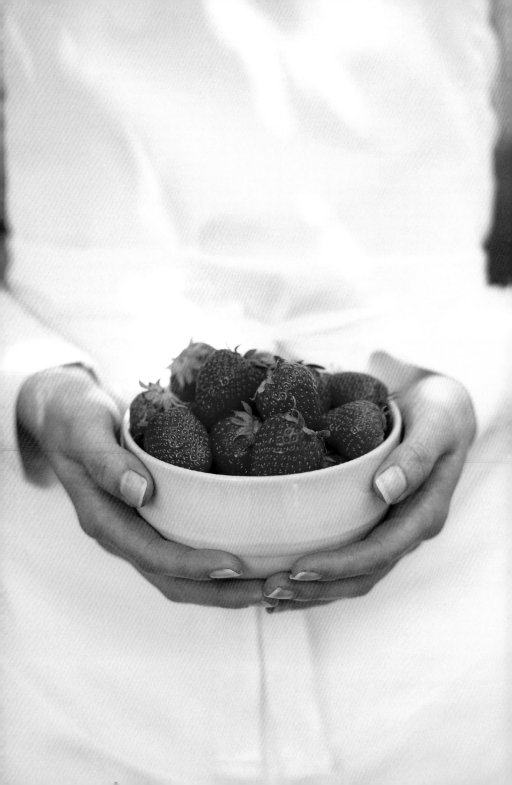

## eye opener

Both carrot and fennel are effective detoxifiers and good for restoring fluid balance because of their high potassium content. Fennel also helps to digest fats, which will help out your overworked liver. A glass of this juice should give you an immediate lift and ensure that the whites of your eyes are white, not bloodshot.

3 carrots
1 small fennel bulb

Juice both ingredients and serve in a tall glass over ice with a slice of lemon, if desired.

Makes 7 fl oz or 1 small glass
Vitamin A 61,027 iu • Potassium 1,527 mg
• Selenium 3.3 mcg • Calories 152

## power pack

Carrots, beets, and oranges are all high in vitamin C, antioxidants, and phytonutrients, such as beta-carotene, and they are also rich sources of potassium. A great tonic.

4 carrots
2$\frac{1}{2}$ beets
1 orange, peeled
1 cup strawberries

Juice all of the ingredients together, then pour over ice cubes in a tall glass.

Makes 7 fl oz or 1 small glass
Vitamin C 166 mg • Potassium 1,646 mg
• Magnesium 91 mg • Selenium 5 mcg
• Calories 259

# day 4

**Smile**, because today
is officially your
**halfway** point

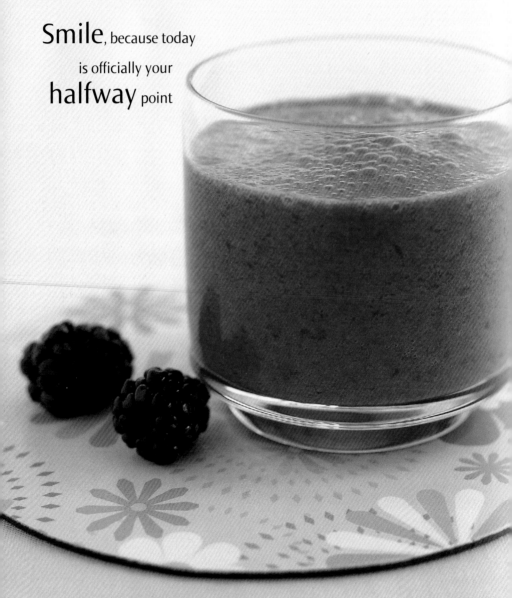

Feeling pretty pleased with yourself? Is it getting a little easier? You really should be over any headaches or other side effects by now, and feeling more energized and cleaner. If you have a good look in the mirror, the whites of your eyes will be brighter and your skin clearer. Keep going, you're worth it.

## ◄ grapeberry cream smoothie

Blackberries and purple grapes contain high levels of fluid-balancing potassium and essential bioflavonoids, while the yogurt with live culture boosts intestinal flora and calcium intake.

1 cup blackberries, fresh or frozen
1¼ cups purple grape juice, or 2⅔ cups fresh purple grapes
3 tablespoons plain yogurt with live cultures

If using fresh grapes, juice them, then place in the blender with the other ingredients. Process until smooth. Serve immediately.

Makes 12 fl oz or 1 large glass
Vitamin C 20 mg • Potassium 468 mg • Calcium 162 mg • Iron 3.5 mg • Calories 200

## on today's menu

### start the day
Spicy Orange Tea (page 80)

### and then on to
Grapeberry Cream Smoothie (page 77)
Red Rocket (page 78)
Mango Slush (page 78)
Control Freak (page 80)
Mother Nature (page 80)

### and wind down with
Any herbal tea or infusion of your choice
2 teaspoons flaxseed

### snack attack
6–8 Brazil nuts plus 2 kiwifruit

## red rocket ▶

Cabbage is a great detoxifier and, when combined with the classic juice combination of carrot and apple, it is excellent for cleansing the stomach and upper colon.

3 carrots
1 large apple
1³/₄ cups chopped red cabbage

Juice all the ingredients and serve over ice with a slice of orange, if desired.

Makes 7 fl oz or 1 small glass
Vitamin C 70 mg • Potassium 1,159 mg
• Selenium 3.8 mcg • Calories 250

## mango slush

Mangos are an amazing source of beta-carotene, apples are cleansing, and cucumber works effectively as a diuretic. This juice is both highly nourishing and system clearing.

1 apple
¹/₂ cucumber
¹/₂ mango, peeled and pitted

Juice the apple and cucumber, then blend with the mango and a couple of ice cubes.

Makes 7 fl oz or 1 small glass
Vitamin C 105 mg • Calcium 38 mg • Potassium 56 mg
• Calories 200

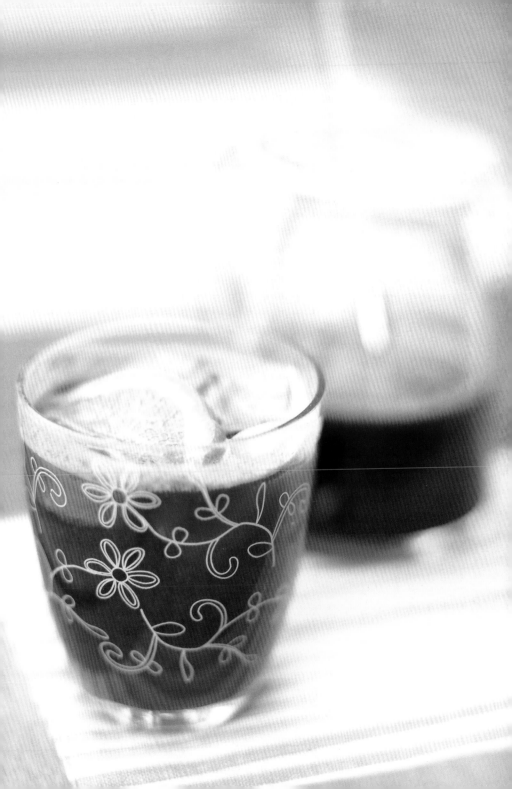

## control freak

As well as being high in immune-boosting vitamins A and C, this juice is fantastic for your digestive tract. The sweet potato removes any toxic buildup and will calm inflammation, and the carrot kills bacteria and viruses. So if you have been burning the midnight oil, combined with eating junk food on the run, this is the ideal juice to put you back on track.

1 sweet potato
2 small oranges, peeled
2 large carrots

Juice all three ingredients and serve over ice, or blend with a couple of ice cubes for a smoother, creamier drink.

Makes 7 fl oz or 1 small glass
Vitamin A 78,357 iu • Vitamin C 200 mg • Calories 358

**FEEL-GOOD FACTOR**
Turn off the television and go to the movie theater or snuggle up in bed with that book you have been meaning to read. It is amazing how many of us will sit and watch mindless television just for the sake of it and not even remember what it was we were watching by the next day.

## mother nature

Celery will help to flush out aggravating toxins and rehydrate the system, while the fennel helps to digest fat and will give your liver a break. Grapefruit is a powerful blood cleanser, but don't drink it with alcohol, because it increases its effect.

$^1/_2$ grapefruit, peeled
$2^1/_2$ celery sticks
$^1/_2$ fennel bulb

Juice all the ingredients. Serve in a tall glass over ice. You could add pineapple and tarragon for more variety.

Makes 7 fl oz or 1 small glass
Vitamin C 54 mg • Potassium 729 mg • Folic acid 28 mcg
• Calories 87

LITTLE HOTTY
SPICY ORANGE TEA
Try putting a few slices of orange, a couple of cloves, and a couple of star anise in a cafetiere or teapot. Cover with hot water and let steep for 5 minutes. Drink freely throughout the day. Alternatively, try Orange Spice herbal tea bags.

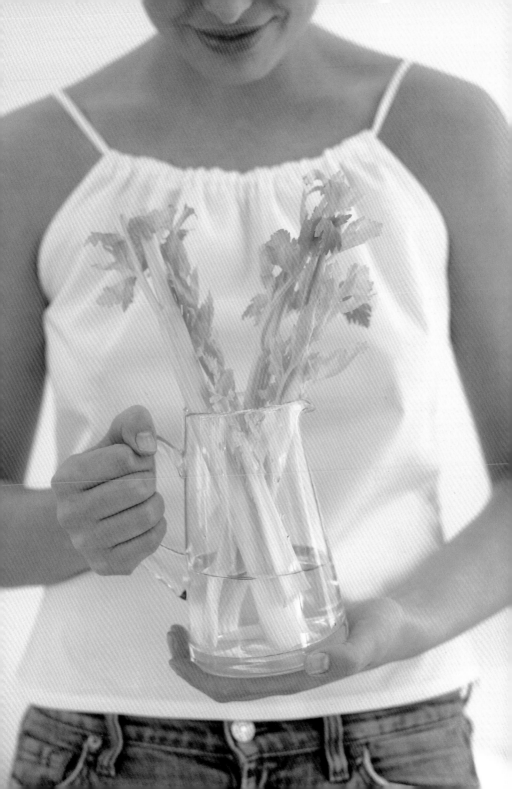

# day 5

Almost there!
Keep up the **good work**
and feel the benefits

Only three days to go! Keep that willpower going and stay motivated. Try on that special outfit; it should be feeling looser by now. Just think how much better it will fit you if you can manage to last until the end and finish the whole seven days.

## ◄ virgin mary smoothie

If you are yearning for a savory treat, this delicious and filling smoothie will hit the spot. Use fresh tomato juice with no added preservatives for a great boost of lycopene.

$^1/_2$ red bell pepper, cored, seeded, and
   coarsely chopped
$^1/_2$ cup peeled and coarsely chopped cucumber
1 large scallion
$^1/_2$ cup tomato juice
Juice of $^1/_2$ lemon
$^1/_2$ avocado
$^1/_2$ teaspoon seeded and finely chopped
   red chile (optional)

Put all the ingredients in a blender and process. Season with a little organic tamari sauce, if desired.

Makes 10 fl oz or 1 large glass
Vitamin C 91 mg • Vitamin E 4.75 mg • Iron 1.2 mg
• Calories 237

## on today's menu

### start the day
Mint Tea (page 86)

### and then on to
Virgin Mary Smoothie (page 83)
Time Out (page 84)
Sharp One (page 84)
Free Flow (page 86)
Pepper Punch (page 86)

### and wind down with
Any herbal tea or infusion of your choice
2 teaspoons flaxseed

### snack attack
3 tablespoons macadamia nuts plus
2 clementines

## time out ▶

If you have been burning the candle at both ends and overloading your system with toxins, give your adrenals a welcome rest and slow down. This juice is packed with ingredients that will act as an effective tonic. Blackberries have a cleansing action on the blood and kiwifruit are an excellent source of vitamin C. The melon is full of beta-carotene and will help rehydrate your entire system.

$^2/_3$ cup cantaloupe cubes
$^2/_3$ cup blackberries, fresh or frozen
2 kiwifruits, sliced with skins on

Juice all three ingredients. Place in a blender and process with a couple of ice cubes. Pour into a tall glass and serve with a few blackberries, if desired.

Makes 8 fl oz or 1 small glass
Vitamin C 215 mg • Vitamin A 4,194 iu
• Magnesium 78 mg • Calories 182

## sharp one

This juice is high in natural sugar, so it's a great one to reach for if you feel your energy levels dipping; it's also refreshing on the palate.

2 pears
1$^2/_3$ cups pineapple chunks
$^1/_2$ lime, peeled

Juice all the ingredients and serve over ice cubes.

Makes 10 fl oz or 1 large glass
Calcium 74 mg • Iron 1 mg • Calories 212

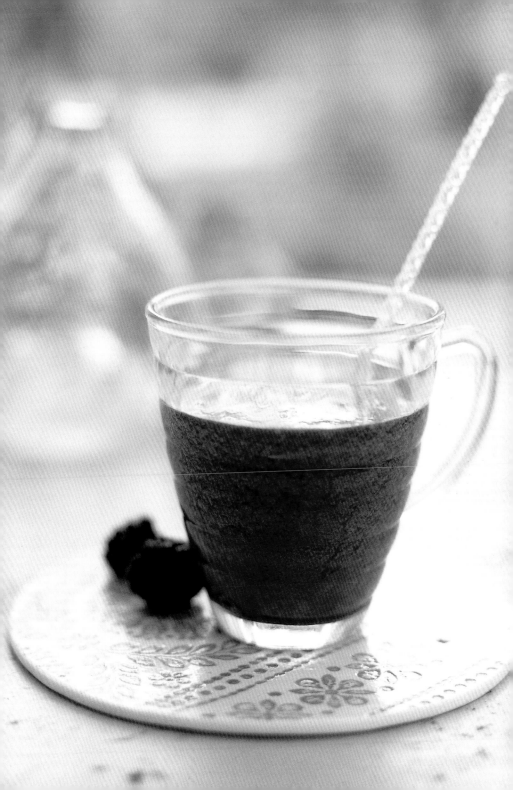

## pepper punch

This is a very-fresh tasting juice that is quick and easy to prepare. It is full of beta-carotene and the bell peppers contain natural silicone, which is a great boost for your skin and nails. Check the vitamin C content—it's huge!

**1 each of red, yellow, and orange bell peppers**
**1 orange, peeled**
**8 mint leaves, to garnish**

Juice all the bell peppers and orange and serve over ice. Stir in the mint leaves.

Makes 7 fl oz or 1 small glass
Vitamin C 333 mg • Selenium 1.5 mcg • Zinc 0.44 mg
• Calories 141

## free flow

When we are stressed, excess adrenalin causes the blood to thicken, which can have a disastrous impact on health if the stress is prolonged. This smoothie is an excellent blood thinner and balancer, because avocado is a good source of vitamin E, which is a highly effective antithrombin, helping to prevent blood coagulation, causing dilation of the blood vessels, allowing the blood to flow more freely toward the heart. It is also vital to pituitary gland function, which ultimately regulates the adrenals.

**3 celery sticks**
**1 cup spinach**
**10 sprigs of watercress**
**1 medium apple**
**¹/₂ small avocado**

Juice the celery, spinach, watercress, and apple. Put into a blender with the avocado and a couple of ice cubes and process until smooth. Serve immediately in a glass and garnish with a lime slice, if desired.

Makes 7 fl oz or 1 small glass
Vitamin C 35 mg • Vitamin E 2.2 mg • Magnesium 70 mg
• Calories 267

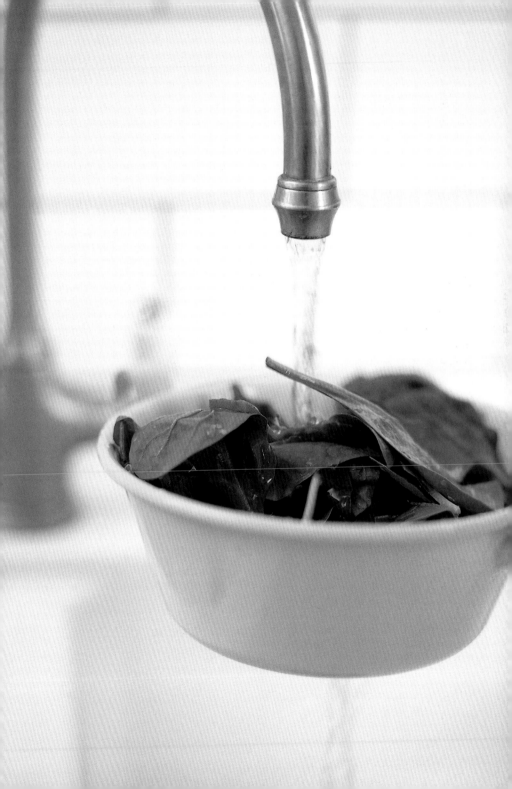

# day 6

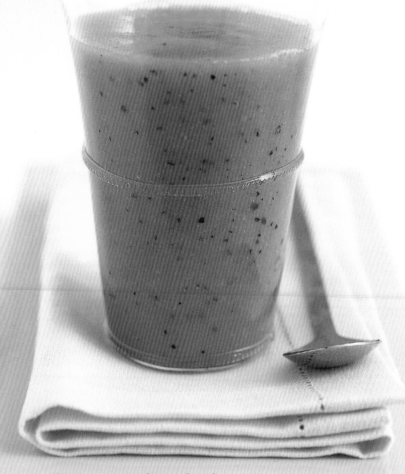

You are within sight of
the finish line, so **keep following**
the diet for a **leaner**, healthier life

So, so close to finishing, so don't blow it by cheating now. You can do this; you might even be enjoying it and your body will definitely be thanking you for the break. Keep yourself away from temptation; it will be worth it when you slip into that outfit or those too-tight jeans.

## ◄ tiger smoothie

Papaya is full of digestive enzymes and is an exceptionally powerful detoxifying fruit. Passion fruit and lime give the smoothie a great zesty taste.

1 orange
$^1/_2$ lime
1 papaya
1 passion fruit

Juice the orange and lime. Cut the papaya in half and remove the seeds. Put the flesh in a blender along with the passion fruit juice and seeds. Add the juiced orange and lime and a couple of ice cubes. Blend and serve immediately. For variation, you can maybe add mango.

Makes 8 fl oz or 1 small glass
Vitamin C 270 mg • Magnesium 25 mg • Calories 135

## on today's menu

### start the day
Rooibos Tea with Lemon (page 92)

### and then on to
Tiger Smoothie (page 89)
Yellow Submarine (page 90)
Melon Berry Juice (page 90)
Blood Brother (page 92)
Super Veggie Boost (page 92)

### and wind down with
Any herbal tea or infusion of your choice
2 teaspoons flaxseed

### snack attack
3 tablespoons pistachio nuts plus 1 raw carrot, cut into sticks

### TOP TIP
The nutritional value of nuts and seeds deteriorates quickly if left in open bags. This is because they have a high oil content, which can easily turn rancid if left for a long time. Keep opened packages of nuts in your refrigerator and nibble regularly.

## yellow submarine

Both celery and fennel are effective diuretics and also have appetite-controlling properties.

2¹/₂ celery sticks
¹/₂ fennel bulb (or try 1 parsnip for a change)
¹/₂ cup pineapple chunks

Juice all three ingredients and serve over ice.

Makes 7 fl oz or 1 small glass
Vitamin C 49 mg • Calcium 115 mg • Calories 144

### THE FIT STUFF

If you are feeling a little tired or lacking energy, then revitalize your system by doing your stretches and breathing deeply, then take your walk at a gentle pace today. However, chances are you'll feel like revving it up a notch. A brisk 15–20 minute walk before your lunchtime juice or to clear the three o'clock energy dip will do wonders; and try to fit in your stretching and toning routine at some point. Hopefully, this new dedication to exercise will become part of your daily life.

## melon berry juice ▶

There is room for a little flexibility here, because it is better to go for fruits that are in season and readily available. Melon is highly hydrating, so it's great after exercise, when fluid replacement is a priority.

2 cups canteloupe, honeydew, or
    watermelon chunks
1 cup strawberries, raspberries, or
    pitted cherries

Juice both ingredients and serve over ice cubes.

Makes 12 fl oz or 1 large glass
Iron 1.8 mg • Calcium 52 mg • Calories 125

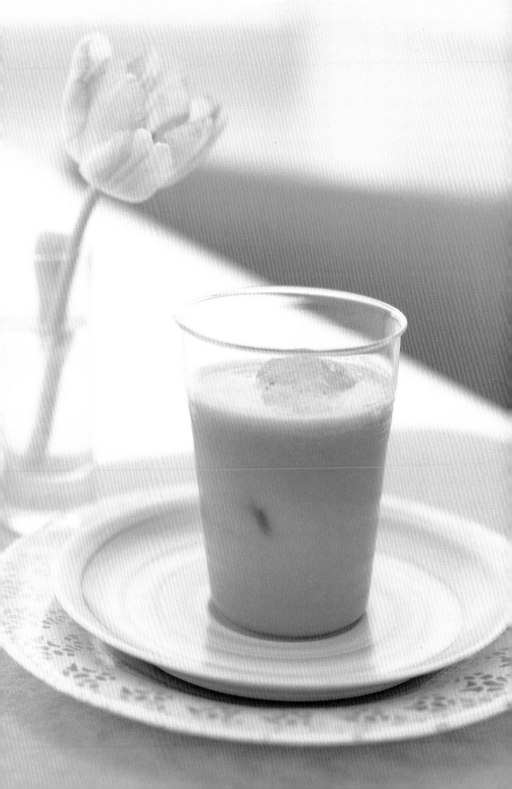

# blood brother

This rich and sweet juice is a great blood restorer and liver regenerator. This is important, because if the liver is overtaxed because of having to deal with harmful substances, such as alcohol, it won't be able to effectively cleanse and purify the blood. This will leave the blood full of potentially harmful toxins, which will be circulated around the body.

²/₃ cup red grapes
2 beets
2 small plums

Juice all three ingredients and serve over ice cubes.

Makes 7 fl oz or 1 small glass
Vitamin C 15.3 mg • Potassium 611 mg
• Folic acid 51 mcg • Calories 143

# super veggie boost juice

This bright green juice is a fantastic way to benefit from a magnificent seven different vegetables. Sipped slowly, it should sustain you and will definitely cleanse your system.

2 carrots
1 green bell pepper, seeded
2 cups spinach
¹/₂ onion
2¹/₂ celery sticks
2 cups cucumber chunks
1 tomato

Juice everything and serve immediately. If you want to vary the drink, after juicing, put it into a blender with half an avocado for a power-packed super smoothie.

Makes 7 fl oz or 1 small glass
Vitamin C 210 mg • Potassium 2,130 mg
• Selenium 5 mcg • Iron 5 mg • Calories 230

**LITTLE HOTTY**
**ROOIBOS TEA WITH LEMON**
Rooibos tea, sold in larger supermarkets and online, is caffeine-free and great if you miss your daily cup—try adding a teaspoon of lemon zest or a slice of lemon. It's almost like drinking a cup of Earl Grey.

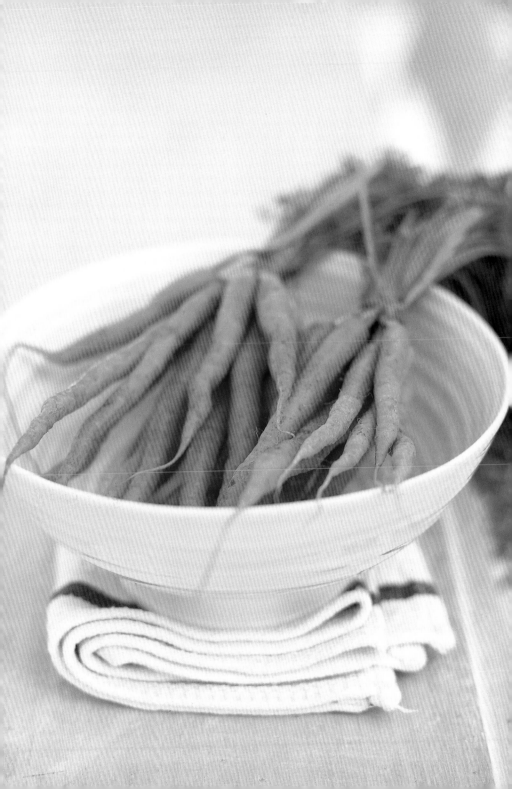

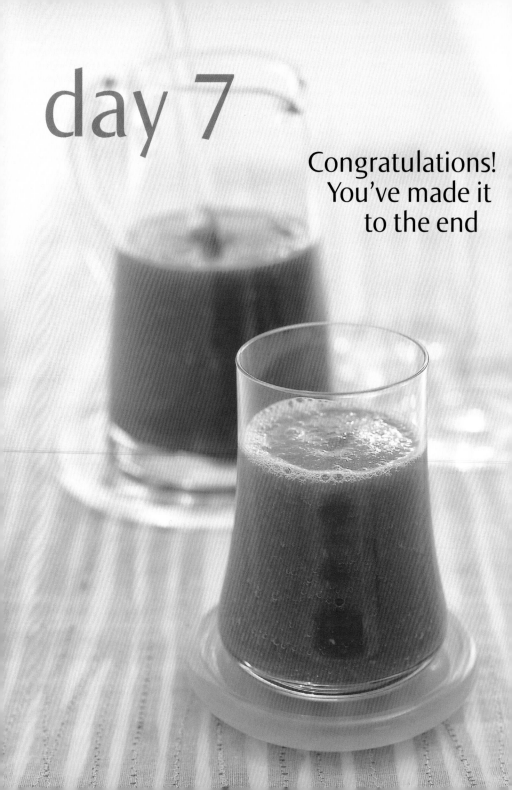

# day 7

Congratulations!
You've made it
to the end

Go and try on that outfit and prance around in front of the mirror. You've almost succeeded—the last day is here. However, remember to be sensible over the coming days. Do you really want to ruin all that hard work by bingeing? Nobody is expecting you to be a saint, but moderation is the key to maintaining your new streamlined figure.

## ◄ sour red

This is a sharp refreshing juice, ideal for after exercise. If you like your juice a little less sour, replace the grapefruit with orange and omit the lime.

$^1/_2$ papaya
$^1/_2$ grapefruit, peeled
1 cup raspberries, fresh or frozen
$^1/_2$ lime

Either juice all the ingredients and serve over ice, or for a variation, juice the grapefruit and lime and process in a blender with the papaya and raspberries.

Makes 7 fl oz or 1 small glass
Vitamin C 188 mg • Selenium 4 mcg • Zinc 2 mg
• Calories 193

## on today's menu

### start the day
Camomile Tea (page 99)

### and then on to
Sour Red (page 95)
Green Express (page 96)
Jungle Fever (page 96)
Fast Track (page 99)
Smooth Operator (page 99)

### and wind down with
Any herbal tea or infusion of your choice
2 teaspoons flaxseed

### snack attack
3 tablespoons pine nuts plus 3 celery sticks

## green express ▶

A super detoxifier, especially if you've had a few too many cocktails, so keep this in mind if you overindulge in the future. Broccoli is one of the greatest all-round foods, because it is rich in vitamin C and A, magnesium, folic acid, and selenium. It is a great antioxidant and stimulates the liver. Spinach has high levels of vitamin A, folic acid, magnesium, and potassium, and will give the immune system a real kick. Finally, apples are superb detoxifiers.

$^1/_4$ **head of broccoli**
**2 medium apples**
**5 cups spinach**

Juice all three ingredients, alternating the spinach leaves with the broccoli and apple to be sure that the machine doesn't get clogged with the leaves. It has a green but sweet taste, so blend with a couple of ice cubes, if desired. Serve in a tall glass.

Makes 7 fl oz or 1 small glass
Vitamin A 18,948 iu • Vitamin C 162 mg
• Magnesium 155 mg • Potassium 1,527 mg
• Selenium 2.5 mcg • Folic acid 270 mcg
• Calories 230

## jungle fever

Papaya calms the digestive system, cucumber cools, hydrates, and flushes away toxins, and oranges bolster your immune system. With a high potassium content, this juice is a great staple when you are trying to lose weight.

**1 small papaya**
**2 oranges**
$^1/_2$ **cucumber**

Peel and seed the papaya, and juice along with the oranges and the cucumber. Serve over ice cubes.

Makes 7 fl oz or 1 small glass
Vitamin C 218 mg • Potassium 1,004 mg
• Selenium 2 mcg • Magnesium 51 mg • Calories 184

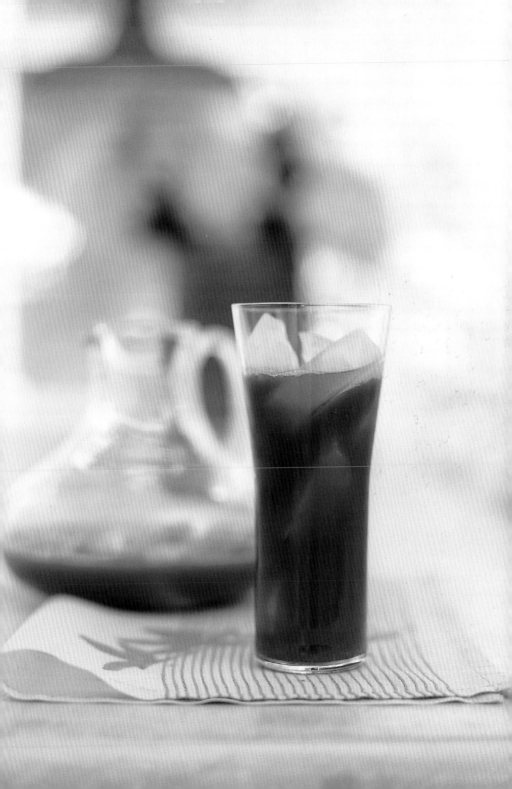

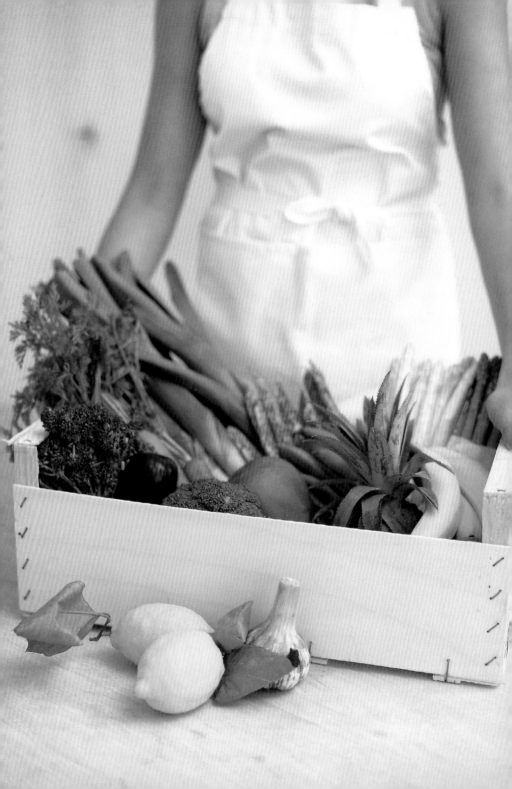

## smooth operator

Bananas are high in tryptophan, which is necessary for the production of serotonin, a chemical that increases your sense of well-being; and because they are high in natural sugars, bananas will produce a sense of fullness.

$1^2/_3$ cups pineapple chunks
1 large carrot
$^1/_2$ lemon, peeled
1 inch cube fresh ginger root
small banana

Juice the pineapple, carrot, lemon, and ginger and then blend with the banana and a couple of ice cubes

Makes 7 fl oz or 1 small glass
Vitamin C 61 mg • Calcium 112 mg • Iron 1.75 mg • Calories 302

## fast track

Before you pull a face, this juice is surprisingly sweet and a great intestinal cleanser due to the cabbage content.

$3^1/_2$ cups chopped red cabbage
1 orange, peeled
$^1/_2$ cup red grapes

Juice all three ingredients together and when ready to drink, serve over ice cubes, or process in a blender with a couple of ice cubes for a more creamy drink.

Makes 7 fl oz or 1 small glass
Vitamin C 247mg • Calcium 253.75 mg • Magnesium 48 mg • Iron 1.45 mg • Calories 302

## LITTLE HOTTY
### CAMOMILE TEA

Put 1–2 tablespoons dried camomile flowers in a cafetiere or teapot, cover with boiling water, and steep for 5 minutes. Be aware: This infusion is very calming.

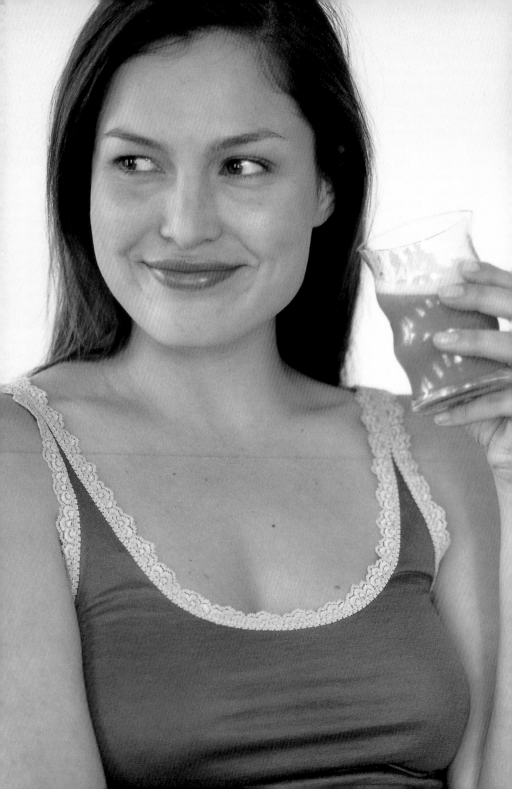

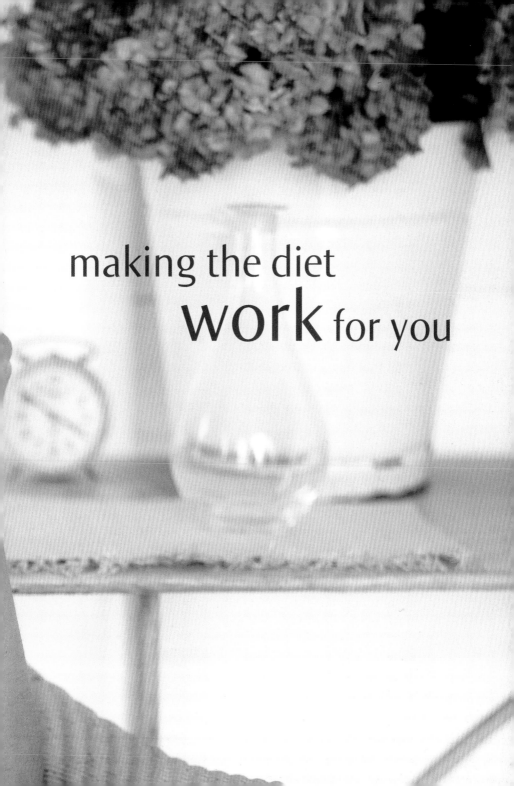

making the diet
**work** for you

# the weekend weight-loss plan

This is the perfect plan if you have a busy **lifestyle** and have to **socialize** during the working week.
If you followed this suggested **routine** for one month, you could **easily** lose 7 to 14 pounds.

Another option is to juice-fast one day a week as a way of maintaining your weight and keeping your system nourished and clean. The weekly menu below will give you an idea of the type of diet you should be following. I have allowed for a little alcohol in the evenings, but ideally you should stick to water and herbal teas.

## weekend-only diet plan

|  | MONDAY | TUESDAY | WEDNESDAY |
|---|---|---|---|
| BREAKFAST | Oatmeal made with soy milk and 1 fresh apricot and walnuts | Large bowl plain yogurt with mixed berries and slivered almonds | 2 poached eggs on 1 slice rye toast with 1 sliced raw tomato |
| SNACK | Seeds | Apple | Walnuts |
| LUNCH | Avocado, tuna, onion, lettuce, and tomatoes | Chicken salad sandwich | Vegetable soup with whole-wheat roll |
| SNACK | Banana | Seeds | Fresh juice |
| DINNER | Chicken tandoori with cucumber-yogurt sauce and vegetables, 1 small beer | Gazpacho, scallops, asparagus, and green beans, garlic, 1 glass white wine | Broiled salmon with selection of vegetables, 1 glass rosé wine |

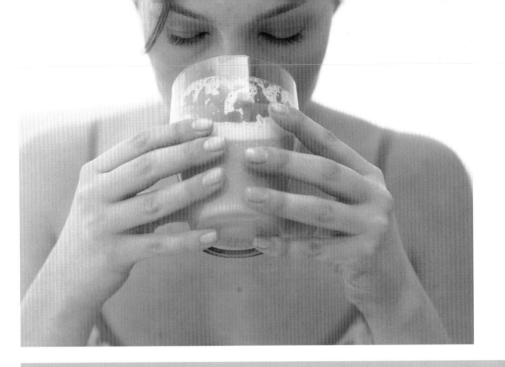

| THURSDAY | FRIDAY | SATURDAY | SUNDAY |
|---|---|---|---|
| Sugar-free muesli or granola with fresh strawberries | Any of the smoothies in this book with 1 apple | Lean Green (page 60)<br><br>Flat Belly Berry (page 59) | Time Bomb (page 66)<br><br>Spicy Lemonade (page 69) |
| Pear | Oatcake crackers, tahini | Seeds | Macadamia nuts |
| Roasted vegetables with cod fillet | Broiled sardines with salad | Chile Orange (page 62) | Ruby Smoothie (page 66) |
| Orange | Pistachios | Spicy Pear (page 60) | Invigor8 (page 69) |
| Sashimi, California rolls, miso soup, 2 small glasses sake | Stuffed baked potato filled with guacamole, green salad, 1 glass red wine | Big Red (page 62) | Orange Super Smoothie (page 65) |

**Note** Vary your juice days—choose from days one through seven. Try to stick to one juice from each color group each day.

# the seven-day, one-meal-a-day plan

This approach can work well, because it allows for you to have lunch with your friends, have a meal (healthy, of course) with your family or partner, or just simply help you stay the course on a sensible weight-loss program.

The weight loss will be slower, but you could probably stay on this program for 14 days and then, maybe, if you have more weight to lose, replace just one meal a day with a juice or smoothie until you reach your target weight. Do remember, however, if you rev up the nutritional value of any banana or avocado-based smoothie with added seeds, flaxseed, a plain yogurt with live cultures, or wheat germ, you really do have an excellent meal replacement.

## the one-meal-a-day plan

|  | MONDAY | TUESDAY | WEDNESDAY |
| --- | --- | --- | --- |
| JUICE 1 | Flat Belly Berry (page 59) | Ruby Smoothie (page 66) | Banana Calmer (page 71) |
| SNACK | Seeds | Apple | Walnuts |
| JUICE 2 | Chile Orange (page 62) | Invigor8 (page 69) | Eye Opener (page 75) |
| JUICE 3 | Big Red or Lean Green (page 62 or 60) | Orange Super Smoothie or Time Bomb (page 65 or 66) | Power Pack or Hi Tension (page 75 or 72) |
| LUNCH OR DINNER | Tofu marinated with tamari sauce, ginger, and sesame oil, stir-fried with selection of vegetables | Salmon on bed of wilted spinach with mashed sweet potatoes | Chunky tomato and vegetable soup with navy beans |

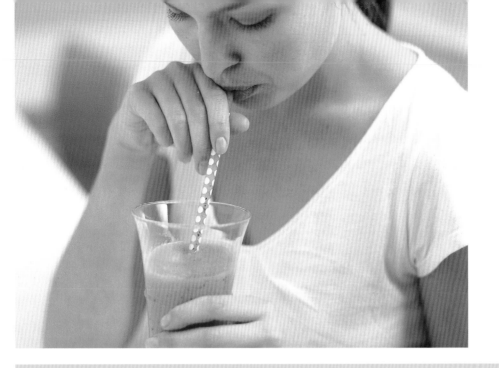

| THURSDAY | FRIDAY | SATURDAY | SUNDAY |
|---|---|---|---|
| Grapeberry Cream Smoothie (page 77) | Sharp One (page 84) | Tiger Smoothie (page 89) | Smooth Operator (page 99) |
| Pear | 2 clementines | Pumpkin seeds | Carrot and celery sticks |
| Control Freak (page 80) | Time Out (page 84) | Blood Brother (page 92) | Green Express (page 96) |
| Mango Slush or Mother Nature (page 78 or 80) | Free Flow or Virgin Mary Smoothie (page 86 or 83) | Super Veggie Boost or Yellow Submarine (page 92 or 90) | Sour Red or Jungle Fever (page 95 or 96) |
| Shrimp and lentil curry with brown rice and spinach | Bowl of vegetarian chili served with iceberg lettuce | Chicken breast poached in stock and fresh tarragon served with broccoli and carrots | Either canned or fresh tuna and avocado salad with arugula, scallions, and cherry tomatoes |

**Note** Remember with both these adaptations, you should still avoid caffeine, refined carbohydrates, and processed foods, minimize salt in-take, drink plenty of water, and stick to the exercise routine previously recommended.

# keeping the weight off

By now you've managed to lose up to 7 pounds in seven days.
Wouldn't it be **nice** to **not** have to do anything so drastic ever again?

## coming down from the diet

Before we deal with that topic, let's get you through the first couple of days after the diet. I would suggest reintroducing solid food carefully.

### On the first day after the diet

**Breakfast** Have either a small bowl of oatmeal with a little fresh fruit, a plain yogurt with live cultures plus chopped pear and walnuts, or if you desire, one of the smoothies with added psyllium husks or flaxseed.

**Snack** Have either a handful of seeds or a banana.

**Lunch** Try steamed vegetables with brown rice, drizzled with a sesame oil and tamari dressing.

**Snack** Have either a juice or some crudités with tahini dip.

**Dinner** Try a large salad with avocado and sunflower seeds.

### On the second day after the diet

**Breakfast** Eat two poached eggs on rye toast or one of the above options.

**Snack** Plain yogurt with live cultures plus honey and berries makes a nutritious snack.

**Lunch** Baked sweet potato with tomato and onion salad will fill the lunchtime gap.

**Snack** A juice or smoothie will help you over the mid-afternoon slump in energy.

**Dinner** A broiled salmon steak with broccoli and green beans is a healthy option.

If you follow the rules outlined in the preparation phase of the diet, combined with regular exercise, you'll stay trim. If you do succumb to the odd few glasses of wine or bar of chocolate, simply replace a couple of meals with a delicious and healthy juice or smoothie to get you back on the right track.

## i still need to lose more weight

Look at the two alternative systems and pick either the One-Meal-a-Day Plan or the Weekend Weight-Loss Plan. This will allow for you to carry on losing weight while still getting the correct balance of nutrients to keep you fit and healthy. Long-term weight control and good health depend on the following:

**Waving good-bye to:**
* Refined carbohydrates and processed foods
* Carbonated and other soft drinks and commercially prepared juices
* Caffeine-laden coffee and tea
* Hydrogenated and trans fats; don't fry food
* Salty snacks and overly salted food
* Sedentary lifestyle

**Continuing with:**
* Whole grains and dried beans and other legumes
* Plenty of fresh fruits and vegetables; aim to eat at least 50 percent raw and rev up your phytonutrient quota by having a daily power-packed juice
* High-quality protein: lean poultry and game, organic meat, fish and shellfish, free-range eggs, and occasional small portions cheese
* Plain yogurt with live cultures
* Healthy cold-pressed oils, such as olive, flaxseed, and hemp
* Herbal teas and plenty of water
* Limited alcohol consumption—ideally the occasional glass of organic red wine
* Continue to take supplements for optimum health
* 30 minutes of cardiovascular exercise and stretching daily
* Strengthening routine at least three times per week

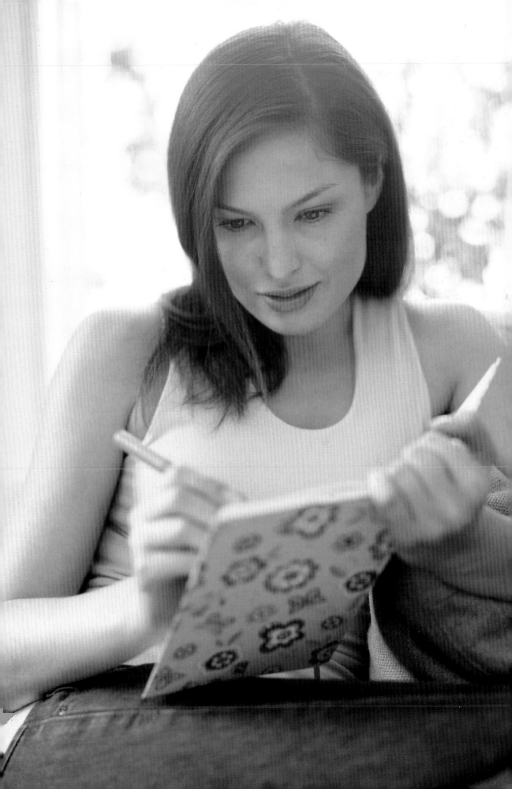

# eating out & socializing

Having a **meal out** should not be a problem; just don't be afraid to ask **questions** and state your preferences— restaurants are used to this.

## basic guidelines

* Be careful with commercial salad dressing, maybe opt for lemon juice and olive oil instead.
* Say no to croutons and the bread basket.
* Ask for your main meal to be broiled, steamed, or poached. Bulk up by asking for extra portions of vegetables or a side salad.

* Have water with your meal and don't add loads of hidden calories by consuming high levels of alcohol—a large glass of wine is around 100 calories.
* If you are going out for a meal, keep in mind that certain types of restaurants are better than others; in general, avoid fast-food outlets.
* Food is better eaten slowly and digested properly.

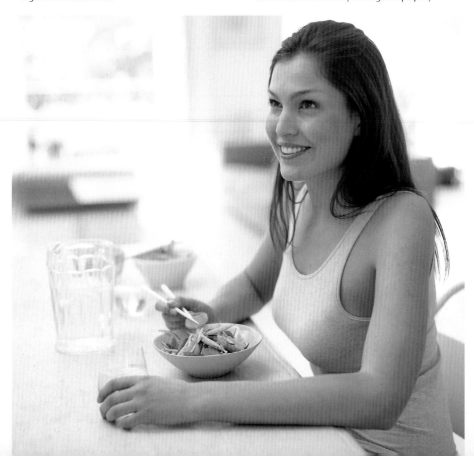

# good menu choices

| RESTAURANT | APPETIZER | MAIN | VEGETABLES |
|---|---|---|---|
| ITALIAN | Antipasto plate, grilled calamari, shrimp in garlic, prosciutto with Parmesan, carpaccio | Broiled chicken, fish, steak, veal cutlets, chicken piccata | Salad, zucchini, eggplant, bell peppers |
| MEXICAN | Avocado salad, black bean and corn salad, Mexican ceviche | Soft corn taco filled with chicken, shrimp, or fish; grilled chicken, shrimp, or veggie fajita made with corn tortilla | Grilled tomatillo salsa, sautéed vegetables, such as summer squash, onions, and bell peppers |
| CHINESE (Ask for no sugar or MSG in sauces) | Chicken or shrimp dumplings | Steamed fish or Peking duck without pancakes | Stir-fries with snow peas, ginger, bean sprouts, bok choy |
| JAPANESE | Sashimi (raw fish), miso soup | Meat or fish Teppenyaki, tofu | Grilled vegetables |
| FRENCH | Asparagus (ask for a lemon and oil dressing instead of Hollandaise), steamed mussels, oysters | Poached salmon, Bouillabaisse, chicken, broiled steak or lamb | Mixed vegetables or green salad |
| SPANISH | Gazpacho, mushrooms in garlic, fresh anchovies, shrimp, scallops wrapped in bacon | Broiled fish, squid, meat—don't load up on paella | Big mixed salads, green beans with garlic |
| THAI | Chicken soup with coconut, or ask for it to be made with shrimp | Most dishes made with coconut and fresh Thai curry pastes—ask for no sugar to be added | Amazing salads with a spicy kick—watch out for added noodles |
| INDIAN | Chicken tikka, tandoori chicken, or shrimp | Most curries with meat or fish but limit potatoes and rice, spinach with paneer. No naan or poppadums | Cucumber-yogurt sauce (raita), salad |

# index

# acknowledgments

**Executive Editor** Nicola Hill
**Editor** Emma Pattison
**Executive Art Editor** Penny Stock
**Senior Production Controller** Manjit Sihra
**Photographer** Janine Hosegood
**Stylist** Rachel Jukes
**Model** Bailee Roup
**Home Economists** Mary Wall and Carol Tennant

The author and publisher would like to thank PPL (tel 01159 608646, www.superjuicer.co.uk) for the loan of their Superjuicer, and www.ukjuicers.com for the loan of their juicer.